The R.E.S.T.O.R.E. MILA Series

Volume 4

Chronic Is Not Forever

The RESTORE MILA Protocol for Systemic Healing

Christopher Thoma, DC

307 Longevity

1120 Beck Ave. Cody, WY 82414

Part of the R.E.S.T.O.R.E. MILA Series: Volume 4

ISBN: 978-1-971449-04-3

Published by 307 Longevity

1120 Beck Ave. Cody, WY 82414

Printed in the United States of America

First Edition

Medical Disclaimer

The information presented in this book is for educational purposes only and is not intended as medical advice, diagnosis, or treatment. The content should not be used as a substitute for consultation with a qualified healthcare provider.

The patient stories shared throughout this book are composite narratives created from the author's clinical experiences. Names, identifying details, and circumstances have been changed or combined to protect patient privacy. Any resemblance to specific individuals is coincidental. These narratives are presented to illustrate common patterns observed in clinical practice, not to represent actual patients.

Always consult with your physician or other qualified healthcare provider before making changes to your diet, exercise, supplements, or medications. Individual results may vary, and what works for one person may not be appropriate for another.

Dedication

To my patients, who have taught me more than any textbook ever could. Your courage in the face of chronic illness, your persistence when conventional answers failed, and your willingness to partner with me in exploring a different path - this book exists because of you.

To the mentors and colleagues who shaped my understanding of functional medicine and the body's remarkable capacity to heal. Your wisdom lives in these pages.

To Ashley and Autymn, whose dedication to our patients makes everything we do possible. Your care and commitment are woven into every success story in this practice.

And to my family - Jennifer, Casper, and Sadie - who give meaning to all of it. Your patience during late nights of writing, your support through the challenges of building a practice, and your love that sustains me daily. This work is for you, and because of you.

Contents

Preface

The question that haunts modern medicine is deceptively simple: Why are we getting sicker?

We have more doctors, more hospitals, more medications, and more diagnostic technology than at any point in human history. We spend over four trillion dollars annually on healthcare in the United States alone.[1] Yet chronic disease rates continue their relentless climb. Six in ten American adults now live with at least one chronic condition. Four in ten manage two or more.[2] Autoimmune diseases have tripled in the past fifty years.[3] Type 2 diabetes, once called "adult-onset," now appears in children.[4] Alzheimer's disease, virtually unknown before 1900, is projected to affect thirteen million Americans by 2050.[5]

Something is fundamentally wrong. Not with individual treatments or specific medications, but with the entire framework through which we understand and address chronic illness.

This book represents the culmination of a journey that began with frustration and evolved into revelation. After over a decade of clinical practice, multiple advanced degrees, and hundreds of complex patient cases, I kept encountering the same pattern: patients with diabetes who also had heart disease, autoimmune conditions, chronic fatigue, and cognitive decline. Patients whose medication lists grew longer while their quality of life grew shorter. Patients who had been told their conditions were separate, unrelated problems requiring separate specialists and separate treatments - yet who clearly suffered from something unified, something systematic, something that conventional medicine refused to see.

The breakthrough came when I stopped looking at diseases and started looking at terrain. The breakthrough came when I recognized that the body does not randomly develop seven different conditions - it develops one pattern of dysfunction that manifests differently depending on genetic vulnerabilities and environmental exposures. The breakthrough came when I understood that diabetes, cardiovascular disease, autoimmune conditions, neurological decline, and chronic fatigue are not separate diseases at all. They are different expressions of the same underlying collapse.

That collapse has a name: MILA dysfunction. MILA - the Mitochondrial-Immune-Lymphatic Axis - represents the three interconnected systems that determine whether your body maintains health or descends into chronic disease. When mitochondria produce abundant energy, when the immune system responds intelligently to genuine threats while tolerating harmless substances, when the lymphatic system efficiently clears metabolic waste - health is the natural result.[6] When these systems fail, when the axis collapses, disease becomes inevitable. Not one disease, but many. Not random, but predictable.

This understanding changes everything about how we approach chronic illness. It explains why patients with "just" diabetes often develop heart disease, cognitive decline, and autoimmune markers over time.[7] It explains why treating each condition separately with separate medications creates new problems while failing to resolve existing ones. It explains why the same person can carry seven diagnoses that conventional medicine treats as unrelated - when in fact they share a common root.

More importantly, this understanding reveals a path forward. The R.E.S.T.O.R.E. MILA Protocol emerged from recognizing that the body heals in a specific sequence that cannot be violated. You cannot restore mitochondrial energy production while the lymphatic system remains clogged with metabolic waste.[8] You cannot rebalance immunity while continuing to pour inflammatory foods into your system.[9] You cannot optimize brain function while cellular energy production remains in crisis mode.[10] The sequence matters because biology demands it.

This book is Volume Four in the R.E.S.T.O.R.E. MILA Series, and it serves a unique purpose within that series. Where Volume One introduced the MILA framework and the protocol, where Volume Two focused specifically on nutrition, where Volume Three addressed autoimmune conditions in depth - this volume unifies the entire picture. Here you will see how the major chronic diseases that plague modern civilization share common origins in MILA dysfunction. Here you will understand why conventional medicine's approach of treating each disease separately has failed so spectacularly. Here you will receive the complete protocol for restoring the terrain that determines whether chronic disease progresses or resolves.

The patients you will meet in these pages are composite characters based on real clinical experiences. Their names, careers, and personal details have been changed to protect their privacy. The medical conditions, symptoms, and transformations described are authentic representations of patterns I have witnessed repeatedly. Their stories illustrate what becomes possible when we stop managing diseases and start restoring terrain.

I write this book with a clear purpose: to share what works. Not theory, but clinical reality. Not promises, but protocols that have produced measurable results in hundreds of patients. The approach you will learn here is not about adding more supplements to an already overwhelming regimen. It is about understanding why your body has failed and restoring the conditions that allow it to heal itself.

My promise to you is simple: under-promise and over-deliver. I will not claim that every chronic condition can be cured. I will not suggest that the path is easy or quick. But I will show you that chronic disease is not a life sentence. I will demonstrate that the body has remarkable capacity for restoration when given proper support in proper sequence. And I will provide you with the specific tools to begin that restoration, regardless of your current circumstances.

To those reading while managing multiple chronic conditions: your diagnoses are not your destiny. The diseases you carry are not random misfortune but predictable consequences of terrain dysfunction - terrain that can be restored. The fog can lift. The energy can return. The body can remember how to heal.

To the healthcare practitioners seeking better answers for their patients: this framework provides what conventional training never taught us. It connects the dots between conditions we were taught to treat separately. It offers biological logic for observations we have made but couldn't explain. It provides a roadmap where standard care offers only symptom management.

The science is sound. The pathway is clear. What remains is the courage to see chronic disease differently - not as permanent conditions requiring lifelong medication, but as terrain dysfunction awaiting restoration.

Let us begin.

With deep respect and profound gratitude,

Dr. Christopher Thoma

Introduction

The One Disease With Many Names

Margaret arrived at my office carrying a cardboard box. Not a folder, not a binder - a box. At fifty-six years old, this former hospital administrator had accumulated more medical records than many physicians generate in a career. She set the box on my desk with a thud that seemed to carry the weight of years of frustration.

"Seven specialists," she said, her voice flat with exhaustion. "Seven different doctors, seven different diagnoses, fourteen different medications. And I feel worse now than I did five years ago when this all started."

I opened the box and began sorting through the stack. The pattern was immediately familiar - I had seen it hundreds of times before. An endocrinologist managing her Type 2 diabetes with metformin and a newer injectable medication. A cardiologist addressing her hypertension and elevated cholesterol with an ACE inhibitor, a statin, and a beta-blocker. A rheumatologist who had diagnosed "possible early autoimmune disease" based on mildly elevated inflammatory markers and prescribed a low-dose immunosuppressant. A neurologist evaluating her cognitive complaints and memory lapses, recommending "watchful waiting" for potential early dementia. A gastroenterologist treating her irritable bowel syndrome with antispasmodics and a proton pump inhibitor. A psychiatrist managing her anxiety and depression with an SSRI. And her primary care physician, who coordinated refills and referrals but seemed overwhelmed by the complexity of her case.

"Do you know what the worst part is?" Margaret continued. "None of them talk to each other. Each one treats their piece of me like it exists in isolation. The endocrinologist does not know that the statin is causing my muscle pain. The cardiologist doesn't know that my blood sugar spikes every time I take the steroid the rheumatologist prescribed. The neurologist doesn't know that my brain fog gets worse after I eat. And nobody - nobody - has ever asked why a healthy woman suddenly developed all these problems at the same time."

She paused, fighting back tears. "I used to run hospital quality improvement programs. I know how the system works. And I'm telling you - the system is failing me. It's failing all of us."

Margaret was right. The system was failing her. But not because her doctors were incompetent or uncaring. It was failing her because modern medicine operates on a fundamental assumption that is demonstrably false: that chronic diseases are separate, independent conditions requiring separate, independent treatments.

The Epidemic Hidden in Plain Sight

Margaret's story is not unusual. It is, in fact, the defining health crisis of our era. We are witnessing an unprecedented explosion of chronic disease that conventional medicine seems powerless to stop. The numbers are staggering. Chronic diseases now affect approximately 133 million Americans - more than forty percent of the total population.[11] By 2030, that number is projected to reach 170 million.[12] These conditions account for ninety percent of the nation's 4.1 trillion dollars in annual healthcare expenditures.[1]

The individual disease statistics are equally alarming. More than 37 million Americans have diabetes, with another 96 million in the prediabetic range - meaning nearly half of American adults have some degree of glucose dysregulation.[13] Cardiovascular disease remains the leading cause of death, claiming more lives than all cancers combined.[14] Autoimmune conditions now affect an estimated 50 million Americans, with incidence rates that have tripled over the past fifty years.[3] Alzheimer's disease, which was virtually unknown before 1900, now affects nearly seven million Americans and is projected to reach thirteen million by 2050.[5]

Perhaps most telling is the phenomenon of multimorbidity - the presence of multiple chronic conditions in the same individual. Among adults over sixty-five, more than two-thirds have two or more chronic conditions. Among those over eighty, four or more conditions is the norm.[15] Like Margaret, millions of Americans shuttle between specialists, accumulating diagnoses and medications, while their overall health continues to decline.

This is not what medical progress was supposed to look like. We have more diagnostic technology, more pharmaceutical options, more surgical interventions, and more specialized expertise than at any point in human history. Yet we are losing the war against chronic disease. Something is fundamentally wrong with our approach.

The Fragmentation Problem

Modern medicine's approach to chronic disease is built on specialization. When a patient develops diabetes, they see an endocrinologist. When they develop heart disease, they see a cardiologist. When autoimmune markers appear, they see a rheumatologist. Each specialist views the body through the narrow lens of their training, focusing on "their" organ system while remaining largely blind to the others.[16]

This fragmentation made sense when acute diseases were the primary health threat. A broken bone requires an orthopedist. A surgical emergency requires a surgeon. Acute infections require targeted treatment. For these conditions, specialization works beautifully.

But chronic diseases do not respect organ boundaries. They are systemic conditions that affect the entire body, manifesting differently depending on individual genetics and environmental exposures.[17] A patient who develops Type 2 diabetes is not experiencing isolated pancreatic failure - they are experiencing systemic metabolic dysfunction that will eventually affect their heart, their brain, their kidneys, their eyes, and their immune system. Treating the blood sugar while ignoring the underlying systemic dysfunction is like treating a fever while ignoring the infection causing it.

Consider Margaret's case. Her endocrinologist focused on lowering her blood glucose, prescribing medications that force the pancreas to produce more insulin or make cells more sensitive to it. But he never asked why her cells had become insulin resistant in the first place. Her cardiologist focused on lowering her cholesterol and blood pressure, prescribing a statin that inhibits cholesterol production in the liver. But he never asked why her arteries were inflamed - the actual cause of cardiovascular disease. Her rheumatologist noted elevated inflammatory markers and prescribed immunosuppression. But she never asked what was triggering the inflammation that the immune system was responding to.

Each specialist was treating a symptom while the underlying cause continued to progress. Each medication addressed one manifestation while often worsening others. The statin depleted her cellular energy production, contributing to her fatigue and muscle pain. The immunosuppressant impaired her body's ability to fight infections and clear damaged cells. The proton pump inhibitor reduced stomach acid, impairing nutrient absorption and allowing bacterial overgrowth. The SSRI disrupted her gut microbiome. Margaret was not getting better because the treatments were targeting the wrong level of the problem.

The Question Nobody Was Asking

"Margaret," I said, setting down her stack of specialist reports, "I want to ask you a question that I suspect nobody has asked you before. Not why do you have diabetes, or why do you have heart disease, or why do you have autoimmune markers. But this: Why did a healthy woman suddenly develop seven different conditions at essentially the same time?"

She stared at me for a long moment. "That's exactly what I've been wondering for five years. They all started within about eighteen months of each other. First the fatigue. Then the blood sugar problems. Then the blood pressure. Then the joint pain and the brain fog. It was like dominoes falling."

"And what was happening in your life during that eighteen-month period?"

She thought for a moment. "I was under incredible stress at work - we were implementing a new electronic records system and I was working seventy-hour weeks. I wasn't sleeping well. I was living on coffee and vending machine food. And then I got that respiratory infection that knocked me out for three weeks. I never really felt the same after that."

There it was - the pattern I had seen hundreds of times. A period of intense stress depleting cellular resources. Poor nutrition failing to replenish them. Sleep deprivation preventing repair. And then an acute illness that pushed an already-stressed system over the edge. The dominoes did not fall randomly. They fell because the foundation supporting them had been eroded.

"Margaret, you don't have seven diseases," I said. "You have one disease manifesting in seven different ways. Your body's fundamental operating system has broken down, and each of your diagnoses is just a different symptom of that breakdown."

The MILA Framework: Understanding the Operating System

The body is not a collection of independent parts that happen to share the same skin. It is an integrated system in which every component affects every other component. At the foundation of this system - the operating system that determines whether health is maintained or disease develops - lies what I call MILA: the Mitochondrial-Immune-Lymphatic Axis.[6]

These three systems form a continuous feedback loop that governs cellular energy, immune response, and waste clearance. When they function properly, health is the natural result. When they fail, disease becomes inevitable - not one disease, but many, depending on where genetic vulnerabilities and environmental exposures create weak points.[18]

Mitochondria are the energy generators within every cell. They produce ATP, the molecular currency that powers every biological process - from muscle contraction to neurotransmitter production to immune cell activation.[19] But mitochondria are far more than simple power plants. They are also danger sensors, constantly monitoring the cellular environment for threats. When they detect danger - whether from toxins, infections, nutrient deficiencies, or chronic stress - they initiate a coordinated protective response called the Cell Danger Response, shifting from energy production to survival mode.[20]

The immune system is the body's surveillance and defense network. It identifies threats, mounts responses, and coordinates repair. But the immune system does not operate in isolation - it takes its cues from mitochondria.[21] When mitochondria release danger signals, the immune system activates. When those signals persist - as they do in chronic illness - the immune system remains chronically activated, creating systemic inflammation that damages tissues throughout the body.[22]

The lymphatic system is the body's drainage and waste removal network. It collects cellular debris, inflammatory mediators, and metabolic waste from tissues and transports them for processing and elimination.[8] When lymphatic flow is impaired - through sedentary lifestyle, chronic inflammation, or dehydration - waste accumulates in tissues, creating a toxic environment that further stresses mitochondria and activates immunity. The recently discovered glymphatic system performs similar functions in the brain, clearing metabolic waste during sleep.[23]

These three systems do not merely coexist - they continuously communicate, with the output of each becoming the input for the others. Mitochondrial distress signals activate immunity. Immune activation produces inflammatory debris. Lymphatic congestion prevents debris clearance, which increases mitochondrial stress. The loop either maintains health or accelerates disease, depending on whether it is functioning properly.

One Collapse, Many Manifestations

Understanding MILA reveals what conventional medicine misses: the chronic diseases that plague modern civilization are not separate conditions. They are different manifestations of the same underlying dysfunction, appearing in different organ systems based on individual vulnerabilities.

When MILA dysfunction manifests primarily in metabolic tissues, we call it diabetes or metabolic syndrome. The mitochondria in muscle and fat cells fail to process glucose efficiently, leading to insulin resistance and elevated blood sugar.[24] The problem is not insufficient insulin - it's cells that cannot use the fuel they're being given because their energy-producing machinery is broken.

When MILA dysfunction manifests primarily in arterial tissues, we call it cardiovascular disease. Chronic inflammation damages arterial walls, lymphatic drainage in blood vessels becomes impaired, and cholesterol arrives to repair the damage - then gets blamed for causing it.[25] The heart itself, with the highest mitochondrial density of any organ, becomes vulnerable when cellular energy production fails.[26]

When MILA dysfunction manifests primarily in immune regulation, we call it autoimmune disease. The immune system, receiving persistent danger signals from distressed mitochondria, remains chronically activated and eventually loses the ability to distinguish self from non-self.[27] It attacks the body's own tissues not because it has malfunctioned, but because it is responding logically to signals indicating ongoing threat.

When MILA dysfunction manifests primarily in neural tissues, we call it cognitive decline, neurodegeneration, or dementia. The brain, consuming twenty percent of the body's energy despite comprising only two percent of its mass, is exquisitely sensitive to mitochondrial failure.[28] Impaired glymphatic drainage allows metabolic waste and protein aggregates to accumulate, contributing to the plaques and tangles associated with Alzheimer's disease.[29]

When MILA dysfunction manifests as generalized energy failure without obvious organ-specific pathology, we call it chronic fatigue syndrome or fibromyalgia - conditions that conventional medicine struggles to explain because it is looking for tissue damage rather than systemic dysfunction.

Margaret's seven diagnoses were not seven separate diseases requiring seven separate treatments. They were seven windows into the same underlying process - a process that would continue progressing regardless of how many medications she took unless the root dysfunction was addressed.

Why Conventional Treatment Fails

The conventional approach to chronic disease focuses on downstream symptoms rather than upstream causes. It asks, "How do we lower blood sugar?" rather than "Why are cells unable to process glucose?" It asks, "How do we reduce inflammation?" rather than "What is triggering the inflammatory response?" It manages manifestations while the underlying disease process continues unchecked.[30]

This approach has several predictable consequences. First, treatments often create new problems while solving old ones. Statins lower cholesterol but impair mitochondrial energy production.[31] Proton pump inhibitors reduce acid reflux but impair nutrient absorption and disrupt the gut microbiome.[32] Immunosuppressants calm autoimmune attacks but leave patients vulnerable to infections and cancer.[33] Each medication addresses one symptom while potentially worsening the underlying terrain dysfunction.

Second, symptom-focused treatment requires lifelong medication. Because the underlying dysfunction is never addressed, the medications can never be stopped. Patients are told their conditions are "chronic" and "incurable" - a self-fulfilling prophecy when the treatment strategy guarantees that the root cause will never be resolved.

Third, the disease process continues to progress despite treatment. Margaret's blood sugar was "controlled" on medication, but her diabetes was not improving - it was advancing. Her medication doses increased over time, and she developed complications despite pharmaceutical management. The numbers looked better on paper while her actual health deteriorated.

This is not a failure of individual physicians or specific medications. It is a failure of the paradigm itself - a paradigm that treats the body as a collection of independent parts rather than an integrated system, which addresses symptoms rather than causes, and which measures success by laboratory values rather than restored function.[34]

A Different Path Forward

The R.E.S.T.O.R.E. MILA Protocol represents a fundamentally different approach. Rather than treating individual symptoms, it addresses the terrain dysfunction that generates those symptoms. Rather than suppressing the body's responses, it supports the body's innate capacity to heal. Rather than managing disease indefinitely, it works toward restoration of normal function.

The protocol is built on a simple but powerful insight: the body heals in a specific sequence that cannot be violated. You cannot restore mitochondrial energy production while lymphatic drainage remains blocked - the waste products of increased metabolism would have nowhere to go. You cannot rebalance immunity while inflammatory triggers persist - the immune system would simply reactivate. You cannot optimize brain function while cellular energy remains depleted - the brain lacks the resources to heal.

This sequence is captured in the R.E.S.T.O.R.E. acronym: Reveal the specific patterns of dysfunction through comprehensive assessment. Eliminate toxic exposures and open drainage pathways. Strengthen immune regulation and resolve chronic inflammation. Turbocharge mitochondrial energy production. Optimize brain function, mood, and circadian rhythms. Repair remaining tissue damage. Everlasting maintenance practices for sustained health.

Each phase builds on the previous one, creating conditions that allow the next phase to succeed. Skip a phase or do them out of order, and the protocol fails - not because the interventions are wrong, but because the biological sequence has been violated.

Margaret's Transformation

Margaret began the R.E.S.T.O.R.E. MILA protocol with appropriate skepticism. After five years of treatments that had failed to help - and often made her worse - she had earned her distrust of new approaches. But she also knew that continuing her current trajectory led to nowhere good.

The first phase revealed the specific patterns of her dysfunction. Her mitochondrial markers showed severe energy deficit. Her inflammatory markers confirmed chronic immune activation. Her lymphatic assessment revealed significant drainage impairment. Most importantly, these findings connected - they told a coherent story of system-wide breakdown rather than seven separate diseases.

The elimination phase was challenging. Removing inflammatory foods meant changing lifelong habits. Opening lymphatic drainage required consistent daily practices. But within six weeks, Margaret noticed something she had not experienced in years: improvement. Not dramatic transformation - that would come later - but genuine, measurable improvement. Her energy was slightly better. Her brain fog was slightly lighter. Her joint pain was slightly reduced. For the first time in five years, the dominoes were falling in the other direction.

By month three, with immune regulation underway, her inflammatory markers had dropped significantly. Her rheumatologist expressed surprise at her improvement and suggested reducing her immunosuppressant - the first medication reduction in years.

By month six, with mitochondrial support in place, her energy had transformed. She described it as "remembering what it felt like to be healthy." Her diabetes medication dose had been reduced twice. Her blood pressure had normalized enough to eliminate one of her three cardiovascular medications.

By month twelve, Margaret had gone from fourteen medications to six, with plans to reduce further as her improvements continued. Her blood sugar was better controlled on less medication than it had been on more. Her cognitive symptoms had resolved almost completely. Her autoimmune markers had normalized. She had lost thirty pounds without dieting - simply because her metabolism was functioning again.

"I don't have seven diseases anymore," she told me at her one-year follow-up. "I'm not even sure I have one. What I have now is health - imperfect, still-improving, but genuine health. For the first time in years, I'm getting better instead of worse."

Margaret's transformation illustrates what becomes possible when we stop treating symptoms and start restoring terrain. Her recovery was not miraculous - it was biological. Once the conditions for health were reestablished, her body did what bodies are designed to do: heal.

In the chapters that follow, you will learn exactly how this healing occurs. We will explore MILA in depth - how mitochondria, immune function, and lymphatic drainage interact to determine health or disease. We will examine the specific mechanisms by which major chronic diseases develop, revealing their common origins in terrain dysfunction. We will expose why conventional treatments so often fail and sometimes make things worse. And we will walk through the complete R.E.S.T.O.R.E. MILA protocol, providing the practical tools to begin your own restoration.

The journey begins with understanding the operating system itself. In Chapter One, we will explore MILA in depth - the three systems, how they interact, and why their dysfunction lies at the root of chronic disease.

Key Takeaways

- Chronic diseases have reached epidemic proportions, with over 133 million Americans affected and costs exceeding four trillion dollars annually, yet conventional medicine continues to lose ground against these conditions.

- The fragmented approach of modern medicine - treating each condition with a separate specialist and separate medications - fails because chronic diseases are not separate conditions but different manifestations of the same underlying dysfunction.

- MILA - the Mitochondrial-Immune-Lymphatic Axis - represents the body's operating system, with these three interconnected systems determining whether health is maintained or disease develops.

- Diabetes, cardiovascular disease, autoimmune conditions, neurological decline, and chronic fatigue are different expressions of MILA dysfunction, appearing in different organ systems based on individual genetic vulnerabilities and environmental exposures.

- Conventional treatments often manage symptoms while allowing underlying dysfunction to progress, requiring lifelong medication and frequently causing side effects that create new problems.

- The R.E.S.T.O.R.E. MILA Protocol addresses terrain dysfunction rather than symptoms, following a specific biological sequence that creates conditions for the body's innate healing capacity to restore normal function.

Chapter 1

Understanding MILA: Your Body's Operating System

Before we can restore health, we must understand what health actually is - and what determines whether the body maintains it or loses it. This understanding requires us to challenge assumptions so deeply embedded in modern medicine that most practitioners never think of questioning them.

For over a century, Western medicine has operated on what might be called the "disease model" - the assumption that illness results from specific pathological agents or defects that must be identified and eliminated. A bacterium causes infection; remove it with antibiotics. A tumor causes cancer; cut it out or poison it with chemotherapy. A gene causes disease; eventually we will edit it. This approach has produced remarkable successes against acute conditions. But it has failed catastrophically against chronic disease, and the reason lies in a fundamental misunderstanding of how health actually works.

The body is not a machine that breaks down when specific parts fail. It is a living ecosystem that maintains health through dynamic balance - and loses health when that balance is disrupted. Understanding this distinction is the first step toward genuine healing.

The Battle That Shaped Modern Medicine

In the late nineteenth century, two French scientists engaged in a debate that would determine the course of medicine for the next hundred and fifty years. Louis Pasteur championed what became known as germ theory - the idea that specific microorganisms cause specific diseases.[35] Identify the germ, kill the germ, cure the disease. His contemporary Claude Bernard argued for something quite different: that the internal environment of the body - the "terrain" - determined whether disease would develop.[36] The same pathogen might cause devastating illness in one person while producing no symptoms in another, depending on the condition of their internal terrain.

Pasteur won. His germ theory provided a simple, testable framework that led to vaccines, antibiotics, and sanitation practices that saved millions of lives. Bernard's terrain theory was largely forgotten, dismissed as unscientific mysticism.

But Pasteur himself had doubts. On his deathbed, he reportedly acknowledged: "Bernard was right. The pathogen is nothing; the terrain is everything."[37] Whether or not this quote is historically accurate, the science has increasingly vindicated Bernard's position. We now know that the human body hosts trillions of bacteria, viruses, and fungi - many of which are potentially pathogenic yet cause no disease in healthy individuals.[38] We know that the same infectious agent produces wildly different outcomes depending on the host's nutritional status, stress levels, sleep patterns, and immune function.[39] We know that chronic diseases - which now cause more death and disability than infectious diseases ever did - cannot be explained by the germ theory model at all.

The terrain model does not deny that pathogens exist or that they can cause disease. It simply recognizes that pathogen exposure is only one factor in a much larger equation. Whether infection develops, how severe it becomes, and whether it resolves or becomes chronic all depend on the condition of the terrain. A robust terrain resists infection, contains it when it occurs, and returns to health quickly afterward. A compromised terrain succumbs easily, fights inefficiently, and struggles to recover.

This distinction matters profoundly for chronic disease. Diabetes is not caused by a pathogen. Heart disease is not caused by a pathogen. Autoimmune conditions are not caused by pathogens - they are caused by the body attacking itself. These conditions cannot be understood through the lens of germ theory. They can only be understood as terrain dysfunction.

The Three Pillars of Terrain Health

What determines the condition of the terrain? Research over the past two decades has revealed three interconnected systems that form the foundation of health or disease: mitochondrial function, immune regulation, and lymphatic flow.[6] These three systems -

which I call MILA - operate as a continuous feedback loop, with the output of each becoming the input for the others.

Think of MILA as your body's operating system - the foundational software that runs beneath all other processes. Just as a computer with a corrupted operating system will malfunction regardless of what programs you run, a body with MILA dysfunction will develop disease regardless of what treatments you apply. You can install antivirus software (medications), delete corrupted files (surgery), or upgrade individual programs (supplements), but none of this will help if the operating system itself is broken.

Let us examine each pillar in depth.

Mitochondria: The Power and Intelligence of Your Cells

Mitochondria are often described as the "powerhouses of the cell" - a phrase so common it has become almost meaningless. But this description, while technically accurate, dramatically understates their importance. Mitochondria don't just produce energy. They determine whether cells live or die, whether they function normally or become cancerous, whether organs maintain health or descend into disease.[18]

Every cell in your body (except red blood cells) contains hundreds to thousands of mitochondria.[19] Cells with high energy demands - heart muscle, brain neurons, liver cells -

contain the most, sometimes over two thousand per cell. These organelles convert the food you eat and the oxygen you breathe into ATP, the molecular currency that powers every biological process. Without adequate ATP, nothing works properly. Muscles cannot contract. Neurons cannot fire. Hormones cannot be synthesized. Immune cells cannot respond to threats. The body does not simply slow down - it begins to fail.

The numbers involved are staggering. Your body produces roughly your own body weight in ATP every single day.[40] A 150-pound person generates approximately 150 pounds of ATP in 24 hours - not through storage, but through continuous production. This ATP is used almost immediately after it is made, requiring mitochondria to operate continuously at extraordinary efficiency. Any reduction in this production capacity creates an immediate energy deficit that affects every system.

But mitochondria are far more than simple power generators. They are also sophisticated sensors that continuously monitor the cellular environment for threats.[41] They detect changes in oxygen levels, nutrient availability, toxic exposure, infection, and cellular damage. Based on this information, they make critical decisions about cellular behavior - decisions that determine health or disease.

The Cell Danger Response

When mitochondria detect danger - whether from infection, toxin exposure, nutrient deficiency, or chronic stress - they initiate a coordinated protective program called the Cell Danger Response (CDR).[6] This response, first comprehensively described by Dr. Robert Naviaux at UC San Diego, represents one of the most important discoveries in chronic disease research.

The CDR is not a malfunction. It is an intelligent, evolved survival mechanism that has protected cellular life for billions of years. When mitochondria sense that conditions are unsafe for normal operation, they deliberately shift cellular metabolism from growth and energy production to defense and survival. This shift involves multiple coordinated changes.

First, energy production shifts from efficient oxidative phosphorylation to less efficient glycolysis.[42] In oxidative phosphorylation, mitochondria extract 36 ATP molecules from each glucose molecule. In glycolysis, only 2 ATP are produced. This seems counterproductive during a crisis - why reduce energy production when you need it most? But glycolysis can occur without oxygen and produces energy faster, even if it is less efficient. It is a survival mode designed to keep cells alive through acute emergencies.

Second, mitochondria begin releasing danger signals - molecules like ATP and mitochondrial DNA fragments that alert the immune system to cellular distress.[43] These damage-associated molecular patterns (DAMPs) trigger inflammatory responses, recruiting immune cells to address whatever threat the mitochondria have detected.

Third, cells become less responsive to normal hormonal signals.[44] Thyroid hormone receptors downregulate. Insulin receptors become less sensitive. This "cellular deafness" is protective during acute stress - it prevents normal growth signals from interfering with survival responses. But when it persists, it creates the hormone resistance patterns seen in chronic disease: normal hormone levels on lab tests, but profound hormonal symptoms because cells are not responding to signals.

Fourth, communication between cells decreases. Gap junctions - the channels through which neighboring cells share molecules and electrical signals - close down.[45] Each cell essentially isolates itself, hunkering down to survive independently. This prevents the spread of infection or damage between cells but also prevents the coordinated tissue function that health requires.

The CDR is designed to be temporary. Acute threat appears, CDR activates, threat resolves, CDR deactivates, normal function returns. The problem arises when threats don't resolve - when toxin exposure continues, when infection smolders, when stress persists, when inflammatory triggers remain in the diet. Under these conditions, the CDR becomes chronic. Mitochondria remain locked in survival mode indefinitely, creating the energy deficit, hormone resistance, and cellular isolation that characterize chronic disease.

This understanding transforms how we view chronic illness. The fatigue that characterizes conditions from diabetes to fibromyalgia to autoimmune disease is not mysterious - it is the predictable result of mitochondria operating in survival mode, producing a fraction of normal ATP output. The hormone resistance seen in metabolic syndrome is not random - it is an evolved protective response that has become maladaptive because the trigger persists. Chronic disease is not cellular malfunction - it is cells responding logically to an environment they perceive as dangerous.

The Immune System: Surveillance, Defense, and Regulation

The immune system is typically described as the body's defense against infection. This is true but incomplete. The immune system does far more than fight pathogens - it monitors tissue health throughout the body, coordinates repair processes, clears damaged cells and debris, regulates inflammation, and maintains the boundary between self and non-self.[22] When immune function fails, disease follows - not just infectious disease, but autoimmune disease, cancer, and chronic inflammation.

Understanding the immune system requires appreciating its two major branches. The innate immune system provides immediate, non-specific defense - it responds the same way to any perceived threat.[46] Macrophages engulf foreign particles. Natural killer cells destroy infected or abnormal cells. Inflammatory chemicals recruit reinforcements and create conditions unfavorable for pathogens. This system is fast but crude - it cannot distinguish between different types of threats or remember previous encounters.

The adaptive immune system provides targeted, specific defense. T cells and B cells learn to recognize specific threats and mount customized responses.[47] This system is slower - it takes days to weeks to develop a full response to a new threat - but far more precise. It also creates immunological memory, allowing faster responses to previously encountered threats. Vaccination works by training the adaptive immune system to recognize pathogens before natural exposure.

Critically, these two branches do not operate independently. The innate immune system activates the adaptive system when it encounters threats it cannot handle alone. The adaptive system, once activated, directs and amplifies innate responses. Both branches must function properly for effective immunity.

Immune Intelligence: Knowing When to Fight and When to Stand Down

Perhaps the most important and least appreciated aspect of immune function is regulation - the ability to mount strong responses to genuine threats while tolerating harmless substances.[48] The immune system encounters millions of foreign molecules daily, from food proteins to inhaled particles to commensal bacteria. It must somehow distinguish dangerous invaders from harmless bystanders - and it must turn off inflammatory responses once threats are resolved.

This regulatory function depends largely on specialized cells called regulatory T cells (Tregs).[49] Tregs act as immune system brakes, suppressing responses to self-tissues, food antigens, and commensal organisms. They also help resolve inflammation once infections clear. When Treg function fails, the immune system loses its ability to discriminate - it begins attacking harmless substances (allergies), attacking self-tissues (autoimmunity), or failing to resolve inflammation (chronic inflammatory disease).

Immune regulation also requires proper resolution of inflammation. Inflammation is not inherently harmful - it is the body's necessary response to threat. The problem arises when inflammation fails to resolve once the threat has passed. Research has identified specific molecules called specialized pro-resolving mediators (SPMs) that actively terminate inflammatory responses and initiate tissue repair. Without adequate SPM production - which requires omega-3 fatty acids and proper cellular function - inflammation becomes self-perpetuating.

The Immune-Mitochondrial Connection

The immune system and mitochondria are intimately connected, communicating constantly through molecular signals. This communication runs in both directions.[21]

From mitochondria to immune system: When mitochondria enter the Cell Danger Response, they release DAMPs that directly activate immune cells. This makes biological sense - if cells are under stress, the immune system should know about it. But chronic CDR means chronic immune activation, creating the persistent low-grade inflammation found in virtually every chronic disease.

From immune system to mitochondria: Activated immune cells release inflammatory cytokines that directly affect mitochondrial function.[50] These signals tell mitochondria to shift further into survival mode, reducing energy production and increasing defensive responses. This creates a feedback loop - mitochondrial stress activates immunity, which releases signals that increase mitochondrial stress, which further activates immunity. Breaking this cycle requires addressing both components simultaneously.

Additionally, immune cells themselves are highly dependent on mitochondrial function. Mounting an immune response is energetically expensive - activated immune cells may increase their energy consumption by tenfold or more. When mitochondrial function is impaired systemically, immune cells cannot generate the ATP they need to function effectively. This explains why chronic fatigue so often accompanies both increased susceptibility to infection and increased autoimmune activity - the immune system is simultaneously too active (chronic inflammation) and too weak (impaired pathogen clearance).

The Lymphatic System: The Forgotten Third of MILA

Of the three MILA components, the lymphatic system is the least understood and most frequently overlooked. Medical education devotes extensive attention to the cardiovascular system but treats the lymphatic system as an afterthought - a simple drainage network hardly worth detailed study. This is a critical oversight, because lymphatic function determines whether the other two MILA components can operate properly.[8]

The lymphatic system serves three essential functions. First, it maintains fluid balance. Blood capillaries continuously leak plasma into tissues - approximately three liters daily.[51] The lymphatic system collects this fluid (now called lymph) and returns it to the bloodstream. Without this function, fluid would accumulate in tissues, causing swelling that impairs cellular function.

Second, the lymphatic system removes waste. Cellular metabolism produces debris - damaged proteins, dead cells, inflammatory mediators, toxins.[52] This waste must be cleared from tissues and transported for processing and elimination. The lymphatic system is the primary route for this waste removal. When lymphatic flow is impaired, waste accumulates in the interstitial space where cells live, creating a toxic environment that stresses mitochondria and activates immunity.

Third, the lymphatic system houses and transports immune cells. Lymph nodes are not merely filters - they are sophisticated immune organs where adaptive immune responses are initiated.[53] Antigens are carried via lymph-to-lymph nodes, where they are presented to T cells and B cells. Without functional lymphatic transport, the immune system cannot mount effective responses to threats.

Why the Lymphatic System Fails

Unlike the cardiovascular system, the lymphatic system has no central pump. Blood circulates because the heart drives it. Lymph moves only when external forces push it through vessels.[54] These forces include skeletal muscle contraction during movement, respiratory pressure changes during breathing, smooth muscle contractions in lymphatic vessel walls, and manual manipulation through massage or compression.

Modern lifestyles systematically impair every one of these mechanisms. Sedentary behavior eliminates the muscle contractions that normally pump lymph. Shallow breathing reduces the respiratory pressure changes that drive lymphatic flow in the torso. Chronic dehydration makes lymph viscous and difficult to move. The result is lymphatic stagnation - a condition so common that it has become normalized, its symptoms attributed to "aging" or dismissed as vague complaints.

The signs of lymphatic congestion are predictable: puffiness and fluid retention, especially in the extremities and face. Dark circles under the eyes. Swollen lymph nodes. Slow wound healing. Frequent infections. Skin issues including acne, eczema, and unexplained rashes. Morning stiffness. Brain fog that worsens throughout the day. These symptoms are so common that patients rarely mention them unless asked directly - they have come to accept them as normal.

The Glymphatic System: Draining the Brain

For decades, scientists believed the brain lacked lymphatic drainage. This seemed to explain why the brain was so vulnerable to protein accumulation in diseases like Alzheimer's - there was no system to clear waste. Then, in 2012, researchers at the University of Rochester made a discovery that revolutionized our understanding of brain health.[23]

The brain does have a waste clearance system - but it operates on entirely different principles than the lymphatic system elsewhere in the body. Called the glymphatic system (a combination of "glial" and "lymphatic"), it uses cerebrospinal fluid to flush waste through channels formed by glial cells surrounding blood vessels.[55] This system can clear even large molecules, including the beta-amyloid and tau proteins that accumulate in Alzheimer's disease.

The critical finding: glymphatic clearance occurs almost exclusively during deep sleep.[29] During wakefulness, brain cells are tightly packed together, leaving little space for fluid flow. During deep sleep, these cells shrink by approximately sixty percent, opening channels through which cerebrospinal fluid can surge. This nightly flush removes the metabolic waste that accumulated during the day. Without adequate deep sleep, waste accumulates faster than it can be cleared, contributing to brain fog, cognitive decline, and potentially neurodegenerative disease.

This discovery explains why sleep deprivation so dramatically impairs cognitive function - and why chronic sleep problems are associated so strongly with dementia risk. It also suggests that optimizing sleep architecture may be one of the most important interventions for brain health. The brain cannot clear its waste while you are awake, no matter what supplements you take or therapies you pursue.

The MILA Loop: How the Three Systems Interact

Understanding each MILA component individually is essential, but the real insight comes from understanding how they interact. These three systems form a continuous feedback loop in which dysfunction in any one component inevitably affects the others.

Consider a typical progression: Chronic stress, poor diet, and environmental toxins trigger the Cell Danger Response in mitochondria. Energy production decreases. Mitochondria release danger signals that activate the immune system. Immune activation produces inflammatory mediators that cause swelling and congestion. Lymphatic flow slows as fluid becomes more viscous with inflammatory proteins. With drainage impaired, metabolic waste and inflammatory debris accumulate in tissues. This accumulated waste further stresses mitochondria, deepening the CDR. Deeper CDR triggers more immune activation. More inflammation further impairs lymphatic flow. The spiral continues.

This loop can spiral in either direction. When MILA function is optimized, it creates a virtuous cycle: efficient energy production supports immune function, balanced immunity prevents chronic inflammation, good lymphatic flow clears waste before it can accumulate, and clean tissues support optimal mitochondrial function. Health maintains itself because each component supports the others.

When MILA function is impaired, it creates a vicious cycle: depleted energy impairs all cellular functions including immune regulation, dysregulated immunity creates chronic inflammation, inflammation and congestion impair lymphatic flow, accumulated waste further depletes energy. Disease maintains itself because each dysfunction reinforces the others.

This explains why chronic diseases are so difficult to treat with single interventions. A statin addresses cholesterol but does nothing for mitochondrial function - indeed, it may worsen it. An immunosuppressant reduces inflammation but leaves the mitochondrial dysfunction and lymphatic congestion that triggered inflammation in the first place. The disease process continues because the root dysfunction - the MILA collapse - remains unaddressed.

Why This Understanding Changes Everything

Grasping the MILA framework transforms how we understand chronic disease. What appeared as unrelated conditions - diabetes, heart disease, autoimmune disorders, neurodegeneration, chronic fatigue - reveal themselves as different expressions of the same underlying process. What appeared as inevitable decline reveals itself as reversible dysfunction. What appeared to require lifelong medication reveals itself as requiring terrain restoration.

This understanding also explains why the body cannot be healed through fragmented interventions. Treating mitochondrial dysfunction while ignoring lymphatic stagnation fails because waste cannot clear. Supporting immune function while ignoring mitochondrial dysfunction fails because immune cells lack the energy to function properly. Opening lymphatic drainage while ignoring immune dysregulation fails because inflammation continues generating debris faster than it can be cleared.

Effective treatment must address all three components simultaneously, and it must address them in the correct sequence. This is the foundation of the R.E.S.T.O.R.E. MILA protocol - not random interventions hoping something works, but systematic restoration of terrain function in the order that biology demands.

Understanding MILA provides the framework. But framework alone does not heal anyone. To appreciate why this framework matters - and why conventional medicine has failed so badly against chronic disease - we need to examine how modern medical practice approaches these conditions and why that approach is doomed to fail. In the next chapter, we will explore the systemic failures of conventional medicine and functional medicine alike, revealing why chronic disease continues to advance despite unprecedented medical resources.

Key Takeaways

- The terrain model of health - which emphasizes the internal environment over specific pathogens - provides a more complete understanding of chronic disease than germ theory, explaining why the same exposures produce different outcomes in different individuals.

- MILA - comprising mitochondrial function, immune regulation, and lymphatic flow - forms the body's operating system, determining whether health is maintained or disease develops.

- Mitochondria are not merely energy producers but sophisticated danger sensors that initiate the Cell Danger Response when they detect threats, shifting cellular metabolism from growth to survival mode.

- The immune system requires proper regulation to distinguish genuine threats from harmless substances and to resolve inflammation once threats have passed; dysregulation leads to allergies, autoimmunity, and chronic inflammatory disease.

- The lymphatic system has no central pump and depends entirely on movement, breathing, and hydration to function; modern sedentary lifestyles create chronic lymphatic stagnation that traps waste in tissues and stresses other MILA components.

- The three MILA components form a continuous feedback loop - dysfunction in any one system inevitably affects the others, creating either virtuous cycles that maintain health or vicious cycles that perpetuate disease.

Chapter 2

Why Modern Medicine Fails Chronic Disease

David had done everything right. At fifty-three, this retired firefighter had followed his doctors' orders with the same discipline he had brought to his thirty-year career. When his blood sugar crept up, he took metformin. When that was not enough, he added a second medication. When his blood pressure rose, he started lisinopril. When his cholesterol numbers concerned his cardiologist, he began a statin. When the statin caused muscle pain, he switched to a different statin. When acid reflux appeared, he added a proton pump inhibitor. When his mood darkened, his primary care physician prescribed an antidepressant.

"I'm taking nine medications," David told me during our first consultation, spreading orange pill bottles across my desk like evidence at a crime scene. "Nine. And I feel worse than I did ten years ago when I wasn't taking any. My energy is gone. My brain is foggy. My muscles ache constantly. I've gained forty pounds despite eating less than I ever have. And every time I mention a new symptom, they just add another pill."

He paused, frustration giving way to something deeper - a mix of confusion and betrayal. "I spent my career running into burning buildings. I trusted the system. I trusted that if I followed the rules, the system would take care of me. But the system isn't taking care of me. It's just... managing me. Managing my decline."

David had articulated something that millions of chronic disease patients sense but struggle to express: modern medicine is not designed to heal chronic disease. It is designed to manage it - indefinitely, profitably, and with an ever-expanding arsenal of pharmaceuticals that address symptoms while leaving root causes untouched.

The Management Model of Medicine

Modern medicine excels at acute care. Trauma surgery, emergency interventions, infectious disease treatment, acute cardiac events - in these areas, Western medicine has achieved remarkable success.[56] The tools developed over the past century have saved countless lives that would have been lost in previous eras. This success is real and should not be dismissed.

But chronic disease operates by different rules. Acute conditions have clear onset, identifiable causes, and definitive endpoints - you either recover or you don't. Chronic conditions develop gradually, arise from complex interactions of genetics and environment, and persist indefinitely.[15] The tools that work brilliantly for acute care fail systematically when applied to chronic disease.

The fundamental problem is one paradigm. Acute care operates on a find-and-fix model: identify the broken part, repair or remove it, restore function. A fractured bone is set. A ruptured appendix is removed. A bacterial infection is killed with antibiotics. The intervention addresses the cause, and health returns.[57]

Chronic disease cannot be approached this way because there is no single broken part to fix. Diabetes is not caused by a malfunctioning pancreas that can be repaired. Heart disease is not caused by defective arteries that can be replaced. Autoimmune conditions are not caused by a faulty immune system that can be recalibrated with a single intervention. These conditions arise from systemic dysfunction - from the collapse of MILA that we explored in the previous chapter - and they cannot be resolved by targeting individual components.

Unable to fix chronic disease, modern medicine has settled for managing it. Blood sugar too high? Take medication to force it lower. Blood pressure elevated? Take medication to push it down. Cholesterol above target? Take medication to inhibit its production. Inflammation present? Take medication to suppress it.[58] The numbers improve on paper while the underlying dysfunction continues to progress.

This management approach has a predictable consequence: patients require treatment indefinitely. David's diabetes medications did not cure his diabetes - they masked its symptoms while the condition advanced. His doses increased over time. Additional medications were added. Side effects appeared, requiring additional medications to manage. The trajectory was always in one direction: more disease, more drugs, less health, less quality of life.

The Economics of Chronic Disease

To understand why medicine has settled for management rather than pursuing cure, we must examine the economics. Chronic disease is extraordinarily profitable - not for patients, who bear enormous financial and personal costs, but for the industries that have grown up around treating it.[59]

The pharmaceutical industry generates over 600 billion dollars annually in the United States alone.[60] The vast majority of this revenue comes from chronic disease medications - drugs that patients take daily, for years or decades, with no expectation of ever stopping. A medication that cures a disease is taken once. A medication that manages a disease is taken for life. From a business perspective, chronic disease represents the ideal market: guaranteed repeat customers who cannot stop buying without immediate health consequences.

Consider the statin market alone. Over 40 million Americans take statin medications daily, generating approximately 20 billion dollars in annual revenue.[61] These patients are told they will need statins for life - that stopping would be dangerous.

Whether or not this is medically accurate (evidence suggests the benefits of statins have been significantly overstated for primary prevention), it is certainly profitable.[62] A cured patient is a lost customer. A managed patient is a revenue stream.

The diabetes market is even larger. Global spending on diabetes medications exceeds 130 billion dollars annually, with projections suggesting this will double within a decade.[63] New injectable medications cost over 1,000 dollars per month - medications that patients are told they will need indefinitely. The possibility that diabetes might be reversed through dietary intervention is rarely discussed, despite substantial evidence supporting this approach.[64]

These economic incentives shape medical practice in ways that are rarely acknowledged. Pharmaceutical companies fund the majority of clinical research, creating inherent bias toward drug-based interventions. They provide continuing medical education to physicians, shaping how doctors understand disease. They advertise directly to consumers, creating demand for specific medications. They employ more lobbyists than there are members of Congress, ensuring that regulations favor their interests.

The result is a medical system optimized for pharmaceutical intervention - not because drugs are always the best solution, but because drugs are the most profitable solution.Lifestyle interventions that might prevent or reverse chronic disease receive minimal research funding, minimal physician training, and minimal reimbursement.[65] A doctor who spends an hour counseling a patient on nutrition and lifestyle changes will be reimbursed a fraction of what a doctor receives for a fifteen-minute medication check. The incentives point in one direction: prescribe.

The Specialist Trap

David's nine medications came from six different prescribers - his primary care physician, an endocrinologist, a cardiologist, a gastroenterologist, a rheumatologist, and a psychiatrist. Each specialist focused narrowly on "their" condition, prescribing treatments without full awareness of what other specialists were doing.[66]

This fragmentation is built into the structure of modern medicine. Specialists are trained to view the body through the narrow lens of their specialty. The cardiologist sees a heart with arteries; the endocrinologist sees a pancreas with islet cells; the gastroenterologist sees a digestive tract with a microbiome. None are trained to see the integrated system - the MILA dysfunction that connects all of David's conditions into a single pattern.

The consequences of this fragmentation are predictable. Medications prescribed by one specialist often interfere with the goals of another.[67] David's statin, prescribed to lower cholesterol, inhibits the same enzyme pathway (HMG-CoA reductase) that produces CoQ10 - a molecule essential for mitochondrial energy production. His mitochondrial function declined, contributing to the fatigue, muscle pain, and cognitive problems that prompted additional referrals.[31]

His proton pump inhibitor, prescribed for acid reflux, reduced stomach acid to the point where he could no longer properly digest proteins or absorb key nutrients including B12, magnesium, and iron.[32] These deficiencies worsened his energy, mood, and metabolic function - symptoms attributed to his underlying conditions rather than to the treatment itself.

His antidepressant, prescribed for mood symptoms that were likely downstream effects of his metabolic dysfunction, disrupted his gut microbiome and contributed to weight gain - worsening the metabolic problems that were causing his mood symptoms in the first place.[68]

No single specialist saw this pattern. Each was focused on their metric - blood sugar, blood pressure, cholesterol levels, symptom scores. As long as the numbers in their domain improved, they considered treatment successful. That David felt progressively worse was treated as a separate problem requiring additional referrals rather than evidence that the treatment approach itself was flawed.

The Evidence Problem

Modern medicine prides itself on being "evidence based." Treatment decisions should be guided by rigorous clinical trials, not anecdote or tradition. This sounds reasonable until you examine how the evidence is actually generated and interpreted. [69]

Clinical trials are extraordinarily expensive - often costing hundreds of millions of dollars for a single large study.[70] This means that only entities with massive financial resources can fund them. In practice, this means pharmaceutical companies. Approximately 70 percent of clinical trials are industry-funded, and the percentage is higher for the large trials that generate treatment guidelines.[71]

Industry funding creates systematic bias. Studies funded by pharmaceutical companies are far more likely to report positive results than independently funded studies of the same drugs.[89] This isn't necessarily fraud - though fraud does occur. More often, it reflects study design choices that favor positive outcomes: comparing drugs to placebo rather than active alternatives, using surrogate endpoints rather than meaningful outcomes, selecting patient populations most likely to respond, and analyzing data in ways that maximize apparent benefit.

Consider the surrogate endpoint problem. Most statin trials measure cholesterol reduction, not actual health outcomes.

Cholesterol is lowered - the drug "works." But whether this cholesterol reduction translates to longer life or better health is a separate question, and the answer is far less clear than pharmaceutical marketing suggests.[72] Similar issues plague diabetes trials (measuring HbA1c rather than complications), blood pressure trials (measuring pressure rather than events), and countless others.

Perhaps most concerning is what does not get studied. Lifestyle interventions, nutritional approaches, and integrative therapies rarely receive rigorous trial funding because no pharmaceutical company profits from them.[74] The absence of large trials is then cited as evidence that these approaches don't work - confusing "not proven by expensive trials" with "proven not to work." Meanwhile, approaches that have been used successfully for centuries are dismissed as "unscientific" while drugs with marginal benefits and significant harms are embraced as "evidence based."

When Alternative Becomes Another Trap

Frustrated patients often turn to functional medicine, integrative medicine, or alternative practitioners hoping to find a different approach. And in many ways, these practitioners do offer something different - a focus on root causes, recognition of the body as an integrated system, skepticism of pharmaceutical-only solutions. But functional medicine has developed its own problematic patterns that can trap patients just as effectively as conventional medicine.

The supplement industry has become a mirror image of the pharmaceutical industry - generating over 50 billion dollars annually in the United States alone, with minimal regulation and even less rigorous evidence. Just as conventional doctors reach reflexively for prescription pads, many functional medicine practitioners reflexively reach for supplement protocols. The result is patients like the ones I see regularly: taking thirty, forty, or even fifty supplements daily, spending hundreds of dollars monthly, yet still not getting better.

The problem isn't that supplements never help - many do, when used appropriately. The problem is that supplements, like drugs, are often used to manage symptoms rather than address root causes. A patient with mitochondrial dysfunction might take CoQ10, carnitine, B vitamins, and a dozen other mitochondrial support supplements. If those supplements are given while the patient continues eating inflammatory foods, living a sedentary lifestyle, and exposing themselves to environmental toxins, the supplements become another form of symptom management - expensive, complicated symptom management that fails to resolve the underlying problem.

Worse, functional medicine has developed its own version of the specialist trap. One practitioner focuses on gut health, prescribing extensive protocols to address dysbiosis. Another focuses on detoxification, recommending aggressive cleansing regimens. Another focuses on hormones, adding bioidentical hormone replacement. Another focuses on infections, treating every positive test with antimicrobial protocols. Each practitioner addresses their piece of the puzzle while missing the integrated picture.

David had tried functional medicine before coming to see me. He'd seen three different practitioners over two years, accumulated extensive lab testing, and added twenty-two supplements to his medication regimen. His wallet was lighter. His kitchen counter was covered with bottles. His health was no better. He had simply traded one form of fragmented, symptom-focused care for another.

The Missing Paradigm

What conventional medicine and much of functional medicine share is a fundamental orientation toward intervention rather than restoration. Both assume that the body needs to be fixed from outside - with drugs or supplements, procedures, or protocols. Both underestimate the body's innate capacity to heal when the conditions for healing are established.

The terrain-based approach differs at the most basic level. It recognizes that the body is not a machine requiring external repair but a living ecosystem capable of self-regulation - if the conditions are right. Health is the natural state. Disease is what happens when conditions prevent the body from maintaining health. The goal of treatment is not to override the body's dysfunction but to remove obstacles and restore the conditions that allow innate healing to occur.

This is not anti-medicine or anti-supplement. Medications have their place - particularly in acute situations or when conditions have progressed to the point where immediate intervention is necessary. Supplements can provide targeted support that accelerates healing. But both should be temporary supports on the path to restoration, not permanent fixtures that patients require indefinitely.

The R.E.S.T.O.R.E. MILA protocol is built on this paradigm. It uses supplements strategically - but always in service of restoration, not management. It sequences interventions based on biological requirements - addressing drainage before detoxification, immune regulation before mitochondrial stimulation, foundational function before optimization. And it measures success not by how many supplements patients take but by how few they need while maintaining vibrant health.

David's Awakening

"So what you're telling me," David said slowly, processing everything we had discussed, "is that my nine medications aren't treating my diseases. They are treating the symptoms of my diseases while the actual diseases keep getting worse. And the medications themselves are causing some of my symptoms, which then get treated with more medications."

"That's exactly right."

"And the supplements I was taking on top of that were doing the same thing - treating symptoms without fixing causes."

"In many cases, yes."

"Then what's the alternative? If drugs don't work and supplements don't work, what does?"

"Restoration works. Not treating your symptoms or managing your numbers but actually restoring the terrain dysfunction that is generating all of these problems. Your diabetes, your blood pressure, your cholesterol, your fatigue, your brain fog, your depression - they are not seven separate problems. They're seven symptoms of one underlying process. Fix the process, and the symptoms resolve - not because we suppressed them, but because they're no longer being generated."

David was quiet for a long moment. "In thirty years as a firefighter, we never tried to manage fires. We put them out. We addressed the source, not just the smoke. Why would medicine be different?"

It was perhaps the best analogy I had ever heard. Modern medicine spends billions managing smoke while the fire continues to burn.

Over the following twelve months, David engaged fully with the R.E.S.T.O.R.E. MILA protocol. The process was neither quick nor easy - decades of dysfunction don't resolve in weeks. But by month six, his energy had returned. His brain fog had lifted. His blood sugar had improved enough to reduce his diabetes medications. By month twelve, he was down from nine medications to three, with plans to reduce further. His weight had dropped thirty-five pounds without dieting. His mood had stabilized without antidepressants. His muscle pain had resolved without the statin.

"I feel like I got my life back," he told me at his one-year follow-up. "Not managed. Not controlled. Actually back. I didn't know that was possible."

It is possible. But it requires abandoning the management paradigm that has come to define modern medicine and embracing something fundamentally different: the restoration of terrain.

Understanding why conventional approaches fail prepares us to examine how specific diseases manifest from MILA dysfunction. In the next chapter, we will explore the metabolic diseases - diabetes, obesity, and metabolic syndrome - revealing how these conditions arise not from organ failure but from terrain collapse, and why addressing the terrain offers hope that pharmaceutical management cannot provide.

Key Takeaways

- Modern medicine excels at acute care but fails systematically at chronic disease because it applies a find-and-fix paradigm to conditions that arise from systemic dysfunction rather than broken parts.

- The management model of chronic disease - using medications to control symptoms indefinitely - generates enormous profits for pharmaceutical companies while leaving patients progressively sicker and on increasing numbers of medications.

- The specialist structure of modern medicine fragments care in ways that miss the integrated picture, with medications from one specialist often undermining the goals of another while side effects generate referrals for additional specialties.

- Evidence-based medicine is compromised by industry funding that systematically biases research toward pharmaceutical interventions while lifestyle and integrative approaches receive minimal study.

- Functional medicine, while offering important insights, has developed its own problematic patterns - excessive supplementation, fragmented specialty focus, and symptom management with natural products rather than pharmaceuticals.

- The terrain-based approach differs fundamentally by focusing on restoration rather than intervention, recognizing the body's innate healing capacity, and measuring success by how few supplements patients need while maintaining health rather than how many they take.

Chapter 3

The Metabolic Diseases: Diabetes, Obesity, and Metabolic Syndrome

Gloria had been told she would need insulin within the year. At sixty-one, this retired school principal had watched her Type 2 diabetes progress despite doing everything her doctors recommended. She had taken metformin faithfully for eight years. She had added a second medication when the first wasn't enough, then a third. She had followed the American Diabetes Association diet guidelines. She had lost weight, regained it, lost it again. And still her hemoglobin A1c crept upward - from 6.8 to 7.2 to 7.9 to 8.4. Her endocrinologist had delivered the news with practiced clinical detachment: her pancreas was failing, insulin was inevitable, and she should prepare for a lifetime of injections.

"I don't understand," Gloria said during our first consultation, her voice carrying the bewilderment of someone who had followed all the rules and still lost. "I did everything they told me. I took every pill. I went to every appointment. How did I end up here?"

The answer to Gloria's question reveals everything wrong with how conventional medicine understands and treats metabolic disease. She hadn't failed her treatment - her treatment had failed her. The entire paradigm through which diabetes is understood and managed is built on assumptions that are demonstrably incorrect. And until those assumptions are challenged, millions of patients like Gloria will continue their inexorable progression toward complications, disability, and premature death.

The Diabetes Epidemic

Type 2 diabetes has become so common that it risks being normalized - treated as an inevitable consequence of aging or genetics rather than the metabolic catastrophe it represents. The numbers are staggering. Over 37 million Americans - more than eleven percent of the population - have diagnosed diabetes.[13] Another 96 million have prediabetes, meaning their blood sugar regulation is already impaired.[75] Combined, this means that nearly half of American adults have some degree of glucose dysregulation.

The trajectory is equally alarming. Type 2 diabetes was once called "adult-onset diabetes" because it rarely appeared before middle age; now it is diagnosed in teenagers, children, and even toddlers.[4] The CDC projects that one in three Americans born after 2000 will develop diabetes in their lifetime.[76] This is not evolution. This is not genetics. Genes don't change in a generation. This is environmental and lifestyle factors creating metabolic dysfunction on a massive scale.

The consequences extend far beyond blood sugar. Diabetes dramatically increases risk for heart disease, stroke, kidney failure, blindness, neuropathy, and dementia.[7] It is the leading cause of non-traumatic amputations. It reduces life expectancy by an average of six years - and by considerably more when complications develop.[77] The economic burden exceeds 400 billion dollars annually in the United States alone.[63]

Yet despite this epidemic, despite hundreds of billions spent on treatment, despite an ever-expanding arsenal of medications, diabetes outcomes continue to worsen. More people develop diabetes each year. More diabetics progress to insulin dependence. More complications occur. The disease is winning, and conventional medicine's response has been to develop more drugs rather than question whether the fundamental approach is flawed.

The Conventional Understanding - And Why It's Wrong

The standard medical explanation for Type 2 diabetes goes something like this: The pancreas produces insulin, which allows cells to absorb glucose from the bloodstream. In diabetes, cells become "resistant" to insulin - they don't respond properly to its signals. The pancreas compensates by producing more insulin, but eventually it cannot keep up. Blood sugar rises, and diabetes is diagnosed.[78]

This explanation is technically accurate but profoundly misleading. It describes what happens without explaining why it happens. Cells don't randomly become insulin resistant. The pancreas doesn't arbitrarily fail. These are downstream effects of something deeper - something that conventional medicine rarely investigates because investigating it would undermine the entire treatment paradigm.

The conventional response to insulin resistance is to force glucose into cells despite their resistance. Early medications stimulate the pancreas to produce more insulin. Later medications make cells more sensitive to insulin. Newer injectable medications mimic hormones that enhance insulin release. Eventually, when all else fails, insulin itself is injected directly. Each intervention forces blood sugar down - and each intervention ignores why cells were resisting glucose in the first place.

Imagine a city where houses are refusing to accept mail delivery. The postal service responds by hiring more mail carriers, then adding trucks, then forcing mail through mail slots with special tools. Mail delivery numbers improve. But no one asks why houses were refusing mail. No one notices that the houses are already full of unprocessed mail from previous deliveries - mail piling up in hallways, blocking doors, creating hazards. Forcing more mail in does not solve the problem. It makes the problem worse.

This is precisely what happens in diabetes treatment. Cells resist glucose because they are already overwhelmed - their mitochondria cannot process the fuel they already have. Forcing more glucose in through insulin and insulin-sensitizing drugs doesn't fix the underlying dysfunction. It accelerates the metabolic collapse that caused insulin resistance in the first place.

The Mitochondrial Truth About Diabetes

Insulin resistance is not a disease. It is a protective mechanism - a logical cellular response to mitochondrial dysfunction.[24] Understanding this transforms how we view and treat metabolic disease.

Recall from Chapter 1 that mitochondria are the organelles responsible for converting glucose and oxygen into ATP - the energy currency that powers all cellular functions. This process, called oxidative phosphorylation, is extraordinarily efficient when mitochondria are healthy.[79] But it is also demanding. It requires specific nutrients as cofactors. It generates reactive oxygen species as byproducts. It depends on proper membrane structure and enzyme function. When any of these requirements are not met, mitochondrial efficiency declines.

When mitochondria can't process glucose efficiently, glucose and its metabolic intermediates accumulate inside cells.[80] This accumulation is toxic. Excess glucose undergoes glycation - binding to proteins and lipids in ways that damage cellular structures. Intermediate metabolites build up in pathways that were never designed to handle overflow. The cell faces a choice: continue accepting glucose and suffer accelerating damage or reduce glucose uptake and preserve cellular integrity.

The cell chooses self-preservation. It downregulates insulin receptors, making itself less responsive to signals directing glucose uptake.[81] This is insulin resistance - not a malfunction, but an intelligent protective response. The cell is saying, in effect, "I can't handle more fuel. Stop sending it."

From this perspective, conventional diabetes treatment is exactly backwards. Forcing glucose into cells that are already struggling to process it doesn't help - it harms. It overrides the protective mechanism that was limiting damage. It accelerates the mitochondrial dysfunction that caused the problem. It explains why patients like Gloria, despite perfect medication compliance, progress inexorably toward worse outcomes.

Metabolic Disease and the Cell Danger Response

The mitochondrial dysfunction underlying diabetes doesn't occur in isolation. It is part of the broader Cell Danger Response we explored in Chapter 1 - the coordinated survival program that mitochondria initiate when they detect threats.[6]

Modern life presents unprecedented challenges to mitochondrial function. Processed foods lack the nutrients mitochondria need while providing excess calories they can't handle. Environmental toxins directly damage mitochondrial membranes and enzymes. Chronic stress hormones shift metabolism toward survival mode. Sedentary lifestyles reduce the signals that stimulate mitochondrial production and maintenance. Sleep deprivation impairs mitochondrial repair processes that occur during rest.

Under these conditions, mitochondria enter a chronic Cell Danger Response. Energy production shifts from efficient oxidative phosphorylation to inefficient glycolysis.[42] Cells produce less ATP despite consuming more glucose. Metabolic intermediates accumulate. Insulin resistance develops as a protective response. Blood sugar rises as glucose has nowhere to go. The pancreas produces more insulin trying to overcome resistance. Eventually the pancreas exhausts itself, and insulin production fails.

This progression - from mitochondrial stress to insulin resistance to pancreatic exhaustion - typically takes years or decades. During this time, conventional medicine focuses entirely on the downstream markers (blood sugar, A1c) while ignoring the upstream causes (mitochondrial dysfunction, CDR activation). Medications successfully lower blood sugar numbers while the underlying disease process continues unchecked.

Beyond Diabetes: The Metabolic Syndrome Spectrum

Diabetes doesn't exist in isolation. It clusters with a constellation of related conditions collectively known as metabolic syndrome - a pattern so consistent that it points unmistakably toward a common underlying cause.[82]

Metabolic syndrome is defined by the presence of three or more of the following: elevated blood sugar, elevated blood pressure, elevated triglycerides, low HDL cholesterol, and increased waist circumference.[83] Each of these markers reflects a different manifestation of the same mitochondrial dysfunction.

Elevated blood sugar results from insulin resistance, as we have discussed. Elevated blood pressure reflects vascular dysfunction driven by mitochondrial impairment in blood vessel walls, compounded by the inflammatory effects of metabolic dysfunction.[84] Elevated triglycerides indicate that the liver, overwhelmed by excess energy substrate, is converting it to fat for storage. Low HDL reflects impaired reverse cholesterol transport - the process by which excess cholesterol is returned to the liver for processing.[85] Increased waist circumference shows where the body stores excess energy it cannot process - as visceral fat around abdominal organs.

Conventional medicine treats each of these markers separately. Elevated blood sugar gets diabetes medications. Elevated blood pressure gets antihypertensives. Elevated triglycerides and low HDL get statins or fibrates. Weight gets diet advice (usually ineffective) or, increasingly, weight loss medications.[86] A patient with full metabolic syndrome might see four different specialists and take a dozen different medications - each targeting one marker while none addresses the common dysfunction generating all of them.

The Obesity Connection

Obesity is both cause and consequence of metabolic dysfunction - a feedback loop that makes it one of the most challenging conditions to address. The conventional "calories in, calories out" model dramatically oversimplifies what is actually occurring.[87]

When mitochondria cannot efficiently process fuel, the body has limited options for dealing with excess energy. It can store it as fat - the safest option in the short term. It can allow metabolites to accumulate in tissues - which causes cellular damage. Or it can excrete it through kidneys - which is why diabetics spill glucose into urine when blood sugar exceeds the kidneys' reabsorption capacity.[88]

Fat storage, particularly in visceral depots around abdominal organs, serves as an overflow mechanism when cells cannot process incoming energy. This is not simply "eating too much" - it's a metabolic adaptation to mitochondrial dysfunction. People with efficient mitochondria can eat substantial calories without significant weight gain because they burn fuel effectively.

People with impaired mitochondria store fuel they cannot burn, gaining weight even on moderate caloric intake.

The relationship becomes cyclical. Excess visceral fat releases inflammatory cytokines that further impair mitochondrial function.[89] Fat cells become insulin resistant, spilling fatty acids into the bloodstream. These fatty acids compete with glucose for cellular uptake, worsening glucose handling. Inflammation increases. Mitochondrial function declines further. More fat is stored. The cycle accelerates.

This explains why simple caloric restriction so often fails for weight loss. Reducing calories without improving mitochondrial function simply reduces fuel availability - it doesn't restore the ability to burn fuel efficiently. The body responds to perceived starvation by further downregulating metabolism, making weight loss increasingly difficult and weight regain nearly inevitable.

What Actually Works: Restoring Metabolic Function

If metabolic disease arises from mitochondrial dysfunction, then effective treatment must restore mitochondrial function - not override it with medications. This is precisely what research has shown, though the implications are rarely emphasized.[90]

Studies of dietary intervention have demonstrated that Type 2 diabetes can be reversed - not merely controlled but reversed - in a substantial percentage of patients. A landmark trial published in The Lancet showed that intensive dietary intervention produced diabetes remission in 46 percent of participants at one year.[91] Other studies have shown similar results with low-carbohydrate approaches, time-restricted eating, and comprehensive lifestyle programs.[64]

What these successful approaches share is not a specific macronutrient ratio or caloric target. What they share is reduction of metabolic stress - decreasing the burden on dysfunctional mitochondria while providing conditions for mitochondrial recovery. Removing inflammatory foods reduces immune activation that impairs mitochondrial function. Time-restricted eating allows cellular cleanup processes to occur. Movement stimulates mitochondrial production. Sleep permits mitochondrial repair. Stress reduction lifts the hormonal burden that keeps mitochondria in survival mode.

The R.E.S.T.O.R.E. MILA protocol applies this understanding systematically. Rather than targeting blood sugar directly, it addresses the terrain dysfunction that generates elevated blood sugar. The sequence matters: opening drainage pathways before increasing metabolic activity, reducing immune activation before stimulating mitochondria, restoring cellular energy before asking cells to perform optimally.[6]

Gloria's Transformation

Gloria was skeptical when I explained that her diabetes might be reversible. Eight years of progressive deterioration had taught her to expect decline, not improvement. Her endocrinologist had been clear: pancreatic function decreases over time, medications become less effective, insulin becomes necessary. This was the natural history of the disease.

"But that's the natural history of treated diabetes," I explained. "It's what happens when you manage blood sugar without addressing the underlying dysfunction. When you actually restore metabolic function, a different trajectory becomes possible."

Gloria's initial assessment revealed the pattern I had expected: markers of chronic inflammation, signs of lymphatic congestion, indicators of mitochondrial stress. Her diabetes wasn't occurring in isolation - it was one manifestation of systemic MILA dysfunction. Her elevated blood pressure, her weight gain, her fatigue, her brain fog - all connected, all arising from the same terrain collapse.

The first weeks focused on elimination - removing the inflammatory foods that were perpetuating her immune activation, opening the lymphatic drainage that was congested from years of metabolic dysfunction. Gloria noticed changes before her blood sugar did: her puffiness decreased, her energy improved slightly, her thinking felt clearer.

By week six, her fasting blood sugar had dropped from 185 to 142. Her doctor was surprised but attributed it to "good adherence" to her medications. By week twelve, her fasting glucose was 118, and her A1c had dropped from 8.4 to 7.1. Her doctor reduced one of her diabetes medications.

By month six, Gloria's A1c was 6.2 - technically no longer in the diabetic range. She had lost thirty-one pounds without counting calories. Her blood pressure had normalized. Her triglycerides had dropped by sixty percent. She was down from three diabetes medications to one, with plans to reduce further.

"I feel like I've been given a new body," she told me at her six-month follow-up. "Not a managed body. Not a controlled body. A functioning body. I didn't know that was possible after eight years of being told I would only get worse."

At one year, Gloria's A1c was 5.8 - solidly in the normal range. She had discontinued all diabetes medications under her endocrinologist's supervision. Her weight had stabilized at forty-two pounds below her starting point. The woman who had been told insulin was inevitable was now medication-free with normal blood sugar.

Gloria's transformation wasn't miraculous. It was biological. Once the obstacles to metabolic function were removed, once her mitochondria had the conditions they needed to recover, her body did what bodies are designed to do - it healed.

Metabolic disease offers perhaps the clearest example of MILA dysfunction because the connection between mitochondrial function and glucose processing is so direct. But the same principles apply throughout the body. In the next chapter, we will explore cardiovascular disease - revealing how the same terrain dysfunction that creates diabetes also damages hearts and arteries, and why the cholesterol hypothesis that has dominated cardiac care for decades misses the true cause of heart disease.

Key Takeaways

- Type 2 diabetes has reached epidemic proportions, affecting over 37 million Americans with another 96 million prediabetics, yet conventional treatment fails to halt disease progression because it targets symptoms rather than causes.

- Insulin resistance is not a malfunction but a protective mechanism - cells downregulate glucose uptake when their mitochondria cannot process the fuel they already have, making resistance an intelligent survival response rather than a disease.

- Conventional diabetes treatment forces glucose into cells that are already overwhelmed, overriding protective mechanisms and accelerating the mitochondrial dysfunction that caused insulin resistance in the first place.

- Metabolic syndrome - the clustering of elevated blood sugar, blood pressure, triglycerides, low HDL, and increased waist circumference - represents different manifestations of the same underlying mitochondrial dysfunction, not separate diseases requiring separate treatments.

- Obesity functions as both cause and consequence of metabolic dysfunction, with excess fat storage serving as an overflow mechanism when mitochondria cannot process incoming energy, creating a self-reinforcing cycle of inflammation and metabolic impairment.

- Research demonstrates that Type 2 diabetes can be reversed through approaches that restore mitochondrial function rather than override it, with dietary and lifestyle interventions producing remission rates of nearly fifty percent - outcomes no medication can match.

Chapter 4

Cardiovascular Disease: Beyond the Cholesterol Myth

Raymond had done everything his cardiologist recommended. At sixty-four, this former construction foreman had taken his statin religiously for twelve years after a mildly elevated cholesterol test prompted his doctor to prescribe it. He had dutifully reduced his dietary fat intake. He had switched from butter to margarine, from eggs to egg whites, and from whole milk to skim. His cholesterol numbers had dropped impressively - his LDL fell from 142 to 68, well below the target his doctor had set. By every conventional measure, his cardiovascular risk should have plummeted.

Then he had a heart attack.

"I don't understand," Raymond said, still pale from the experience, sitting in my office three months after his cardiac event. "My cholesterol was perfect. Perfect. I did everything right. How does someone with an LDL of 68 have a heart attack?"

The answer to Raymond's question challenges one of modern medicine's most cherished beliefs - the idea that cholesterol causes heart disease and that lowering cholesterol prevents it. This hypothesis, despite being treated as established fact, has been seriously questioned by researchers who have documented substantial contradictory evidence.[92,93] Yet it has shaped cardiovascular treatment for over fifty years, leading millions of patients down a path that may not only fail to protect them but actively contribute to the dysfunction that causes heart disease in the first place.

The Real Leading Cause of Death

Cardiovascular disease remains the leading cause of death worldwide, claiming approximately 18 million lives annually - more than all cancers combined.[94] In the United States alone, someone dies from cardiovascular disease every 33 seconds.[14] Despite decades of statin prescriptions, despite aggressive cholesterol-lowering campaigns, despite billions spent on cardiac procedures, the epidemic continues largely unabated.

The statistics reveal an uncomfortable truth. Heart disease death rates declined significantly from the 1960s through the 1990s - a period that preceded widespread statin use.[95] The decline has since plateaued and, in some demographics, has actually reversed, despite statins becoming among the most prescribed medications in history.[96] If the cholesterol hypothesis were correct - if lowering cholesterol truly prevented heart disease - we should be witnessing a dramatic reduction in cardiac events. We are not.

Even more troubling is what happens to patients who achieve their cholesterol targets. Studies consistently show that fifty percent or more of heart attacks occur in people with normal or even low cholesterol.[97] Raymond's experience - a heart attack despite excellent cholesterol numbers - is not an anomaly. It is disturbingly common. If cholesterol were the primary cause of heart disease, this would be impossible. The fact that it happens routinely suggests we have fundamentally misunderstood what causes cardiovascular disease.

The Cholesterol Hypothesis: A Theory Treated as Fact

The idea that cholesterol causes heart disease emerged in the mid-twentieth century, based largely on observational studies showing correlations between blood cholesterol levels and cardiac events.[98] The hypothesis proposed a simple mechanism: excess cholesterol in the blood deposits in arterial walls, forming plaques that narrow arteries and eventually cause heart attacks when they rupture or block blood flow completely.

This hypothesis was adopted rapidly by medical institutions and pharmaceutical companies, despite significant contradictory evidence.[99] Many populations with high cholesterol have low rates of heart disease. Many populations with low cholesterol have high rates. Elderly individuals with higher cholesterol actually live longer than those with lower cholesterol.[100] Women derive minimal benefit from cholesterol lowering despite being prescribed statins at similar rates to men.

[101] None of these findings fit the hypothesis, yet they have been largely ignored.

The most damaging evidence against the cholesterol hypothesis comes from clinical trials themselves. When examining all-cause mortality - not just cardiac deaths, but death from any cause - the benefits of cholesterol lowering largely disappear. For primary prevention (people who have not yet had a cardiac event), statins provide minimal mortality benefit despite significantly lowering cholesterol. People live slightly longer without heart attacks but die slightly sooner from other causes, leaving total lifespan essentially unchanged.

This suggests something critical: cholesterol may be a marker for cardiovascular risk without being the cause of it. Lowering the marker doesn't address whatever is actually causing the damage. It's like breaking a thermometer to treat a fever - the number goes down, but the underlying condition continues.[102]

What Actually Causes Heart Disease

If not cholesterol, what does cause atherosclerosis and heart attacks? The evidence increasingly points to inflammation as the primary driver - specifically, chronic inflammation of arterial walls that creates the conditions for plaque formation.[25]

The process begins with damage to the endothelium - the thin layer of cells lining arterial walls. This damage can result from numerous factors: oxidative stress, elevated blood sugar, chronic inflammation, toxin exposure, or mechanical stress from high blood pressure.[84] When the endothelium is damaged, the body mounts an inflammatory response to repair it.

Cholesterol enters the picture as part of this repair response, not as the initiating cause. LDL particles - the so-called "bad cholesterol" - transport cholesterol to damaged areas where it is needed for cell membrane repair.[103] The problem arises when LDL particles become oxidized or modified by the inflammatory environment. These modified particles get trapped in the arterial wall and trigger further immune responses, creating a self-perpetuating cycle of inflammation.

From this perspective, cholesterol is more like a firefighter than an arsonist. It arrives at the scene of damage attempting to help. Finding cholesterol at the site of arterial plaques and blaming it for heart disease is like finding firefighters at burning buildings and concluding that firefighters cause fires. The association is real; the causation is backwards.

This understanding explains why lowering cholesterol provides such modest benefits. Reducing the supply of repair materials doesn't fix the underlying damage that attracted them. The inflammation continues. The endothelial dysfunction persists. Heart disease progresses, just perhaps slightly more slowly because there's less material available for plaque formation.[104]

The Heart as a Mitochondrial Organ

The heart is perhaps the most mitochondria-dependent organ in the body. Cardiac muscle cells contain more mitochondria than any other cell type - up to 5,000 per cell, comprising roughly 30 percent of cellular volume.[105] This makes sense given the heart's relentless workload: it beats approximately 100,000 times daily, never resting, never taking breaks, for an entire lifetime. This constant work requires enormous energy - the heart consumes more ATP relative to its size than any other organ.

When mitochondrial function declines, the heart is among the first organs to suffer. Reduced ATP production means reduced contractile force. The heart pumps less efficiently. Cardiac output falls. The body compensates by increasing heart rate or blood pressure, creating additional stress that further damages an already-struggling organ.[106]

Heart failure - a condition in which the heart cannot pump sufficient blood to meet the body's needs - is fundamentally a disease of mitochondrial energy deficit.[26] Studies consistently show reduced mitochondrial function in failing hearts. The muscle hasn't structurally failed; it has energetically failed. It cannot generate the ATP required to contract forcefully and consistently.

This mitochondrial perspective transforms how we understand cardiovascular disease. The question is not "How do we lower cholesterol?" but "How do we restore cardiac mitochondrial function?" The focus shifts from chasing a number to restoring the energetic capacity that heart health requires.

Statins: A Double-Edged Sword

Statin medications work by inhibiting HMG-CoA reductase, an enzyme essential for cholesterol synthesis. This effectively lowers blood cholesterol levels. What is less commonly discussed is that the same enzyme pathway produces coenzyme Q10 (CoQ10) - a molecule absolutely essential for mitochondrial energy production.[31]

CoQ10 functions as an electron carrier in the mitochondrial respiratory chain - the process by which ATP is generated. Without adequate CoQ10, mitochondria cannot produce energy efficiently.[107] Every cell in the body is affected, but the impact is greatest in organs with high energy demands - the heart, brain, and skeletal muscles.

Studies consistently show that statin use reduces CoQ10 levels by 25 to 50 percent.[108] This creates a troubling paradox: a medication prescribed to protect the heart actually impairs the energy production that heart function depends upon. The heart needs ATP to pump. Statins reduce the heart's ability to produce ATP. The logic suggests that statins might protect against one mechanism of heart disease (plaque formation) while contributing to another (energetic failure).

This may explain the phenomenon of statin-induced cardiomyopathy - heart failure that develops in patients taking statins.[109] It may also explain why statins provide such modest mortality benefits. Whatever protection they offer against atherosclerosis may be offset by the energetic impairment they cause. The heart is being "protected" by a medication that undermines its fundamental function.

The muscle pain and weakness that affect up to 30 percent of statin users reflect this same mechanism.[110] Skeletal muscles, like cardiac muscle, depend heavily on mitochondrial energy production. When CoQ10 is depleted, muscles cannot generate sufficient ATP for normal function. Pain, weakness, and cramping result - symptoms that are often dismissed as unrelated to the medication or treated with additional drugs rather than recognized as predictable consequences of mitochondrial impairment.

Cardiovascular Disease Through the MILA Lens

Understanding cardiovascular disease through the MILA framework reveals connections that the cholesterol hypothesis obscures. Heart disease is not an isolated organ problem - it is a systemic manifestation of the same terrain dysfunction that produces diabetes, autoimmune conditions, and neurological decline.

Mitochondrial dysfunction impairs both cardiac energy production and vascular function. The endothelium - that critical arterial lining whose damage initiates atherosclerosis - depends on mitochondria to maintain integrity and produce nitric oxide for vessel dilation.[111] When mitochondria fail, endothelial function fails with them. Blood vessels become stiff, inflamed, and vulnerable to damage.

Immune dysregulation drives the chronic inflammation that damages arterial walls. Atherosclerosis is now recognized as fundamentally an inflammatory disease.[112] The immune cells that infiltrate arterial plaques - macrophages, T cells, inflammatory mediators - are responding to perceived threats. When immune regulation fails, when inflammation cannot properly resolve, these responses become self-perpetuating, driving progressive plaque formation regardless of cholesterol levels.

Lymphatic impairment prevents clearance of inflammatory debris from vessel walls. The cardiovascular system has its own lymphatic network responsible for removing waste and maintaining tissue health.[113] When lymphatic flow is compromised, metabolic debris accumulates in and around blood vessels, perpetuating the inflammatory environment that drives atherosclerosis.

This explains why cardiovascular disease clusters so consistently with metabolic disease. Patients with diabetes have dramatically elevated cardiovascular risk - not because high blood sugar directly damages arteries, but because the same MILA dysfunction that produces insulin resistance also produces vascular inflammation and cardiac energy deficit. Treating the blood sugar without addressing the underlying terrain dysfunction fails to prevent cardiovascular complications because the root cause remains active.

What Actually Protects the Heart

If cholesterol reduction provides minimal protection, what actually prevents heart disease? The evidence points consistently toward approaches that address inflammation, support mitochondrial function, and restore terrain health.[114]

Anti-inflammatory nutrition reduces the arterial damage that initiates atherosclerosis. Diets rich in omega-3 fatty acids, polyphenols, and antioxidants consistently show cardiovascular benefits that far exceed those of cholesterol lowering.[9] The Mediterranean diet, for example, reduced cardiovascular events by 30 percent in the landmark PREDIMED trial - a benefit achieved without significantly changing cholesterol levels.[115]

Movement and exercise stimulate mitochondrial production, improve endothelial function, enhance lymphatic flow, and reduce inflammation.[116] Regular physical activity is one of the most powerful cardiovascular protectants known - far more effective than any medication. Yet it receives a fraction of the attention given to cholesterol management.

Stress reduction lowers the chronic cortisol elevation that drives inflammation, raises blood pressure, and impairs mitochondrial function.[117] Chronic psychological stress is a significant cardiovascular risk factor - one that cannot be addressed with medications but responds powerfully to lifestyle intervention.

Sleep optimization allows cardiovascular repair processes that occur during rest.[118] Sleep deprivation is independently associated with increased cardiovascular risk, hypertension, and cardiac events. The heart needs rest to recover from daily demands - rest that chronic sleep deprivation denies it.

These approaches share a common thread: they restore terrain function rather than manipulating individual biomarkers. They create the conditions in which cardiovascular health maintains itself naturally, rather than attempting to force protection through pharmaceutical intervention.

Raymond's Recovery

Raymond's heart attack had been a wake-up call, but not in the way his cardiologist intended. The recommendation following his event was more aggressive statin therapy - doubling down on the approach that had already failed. Raymond had different ideas.

"You're telling me," he said, processing what I had explained, "that the medication I took for twelve years to prevent a heart attack might have actually contributed to it. That lowering my cholesterol starved my heart of the energy it needed to function."

"I'm telling you that's one possibility worth considering," I replied. "What I know for certain is that your heart attack happened despite perfect cholesterol numbers. That tells us cholesterol wasn't the primary driver of your disease. Something else was - and that something else remains unaddressed."

Raymond's assessment revealed what I expected: markers of chronic inflammation, signs of mitochondrial depletion consistent with long-term statin use, evidence of metabolic dysfunction that had been masked by his medication-altered lipid panel. His LDL had been low, but his inflammatory markers were elevated. His CoQ10 levels were severely depleted. His terrain was a landscape of dysfunction that his cholesterol numbers had concealed.

Working with his cardiologist - who was initially skeptical but ultimately supportive - Raymond began the R.E.S.T.O.R.E. MILA protocol. CoQ10 supplementation was an immediate priority, replenishing what twelve years of statin therapy had depleted. Anti-inflammatory nutrition replaced the low-fat diet that had paradoxically contributed to his metabolic dysfunction.

Movement became medicine - cardiac rehabilitation expanded into a comprehensive exercise program.

The changes came gradually but unmistakably. By month three, Raymond's energy had improved significantly. The muscle pain he had attributed to aging resolved as his CoQ10 levels normalized. His blood pressure, which had required medication despite statin therapy, began to normalize without pharmaceutical intervention.

By month six, his inflammatory markers had dropped dramatically. His cardiologist noted that his follow-up cardiac imaging showed no progression of arterial disease - unusual for someone post-heart attack. Raymond's cholesterol had risen modestly without the statin, but his overall cardiovascular risk profile had improved substantially.

"My numbers are different," Raymond observed at his one-year follow-up. "My cholesterol is higher than it was on the statin. But I feel better than I have in years. My heart feels stronger. My energy is better. Everything my doctor was worried about - except that one number - has improved."

Raymond's recovery illustrates a critical point: cardiovascular health is not determined by a single biomarker. It emerges from the integrated function of MILA - from mitochondria producing sufficient energy, from inflammation properly regulated, from lymphatic flow clearing metabolic debris. Address the terrain, and the heart has what it needs to heal.

Cardiovascular disease and metabolic disease share common roots in MILA dysfunction. But what happens when the immune system itself becomes the problem - when the body's defense network turns against its own tissues? In the next chapter, we will explore autoimmune conditions, revealing how immune dysregulation arises from the same terrain collapse and why addressing that terrain offers hope that immunosuppression cannot provide.

Key Takeaways

- Cardiovascular disease remains the leading cause of death despite decades of aggressive cholesterol lowering, with fifty percent or more of heart attacks occurring in people with normal or low cholesterol - suggesting the cholesterol hypothesis is fundamentally incomplete.

- Cholesterol functions more as a repair molecule than a cause of damage - LDL arrives at sites of arterial injury to assist with repair, making its presence at plaques an effect rather than a cause of cardiovascular disease.

- Chronic inflammation drives atherosclerosis by damaging endothelial cells, triggering immune responses, and creating conditions in which arterial plaques form and progress regardless of cholesterol levels.

- The heart is the most mitochondria-dependent organ in the body, containing up to 5,000 mitochondria per cell, making cardiac function exquisitely sensitive to anything that impairs mitochondrial energy production.

- Statin medications deplete CoQ10 by 25 to 50 percent, potentially impairing the very organ they are prescribed to protect and explaining why mortality benefits are so modest despite dramatic cholesterol reductions.

- True cardiovascular protection comes from addressing terrain dysfunction through anti-inflammatory nutrition, movement, stress reduction, and sleep optimization - approaches that restore the conditions for cardiac health rather than manipulating individual biomarkers.

Chapter 5

Autoimmune Conditions: When MILA Confusion Becomes Self-Attack

The immune system faces an impossible task. It must distinguish between the body's own tissues - which must be protected - and foreign invaders that must be destroyed. It must recognize trillions of self-molecules as friendly while remaining vigilant against millions of potential pathogens. It must mount aggressive responses to genuine threats while tolerating the harmless foreign substances we encounter constantly in food, air, and environment. When this discrimination fails, the immune system turns against the body it was designed to protect.

Autoimmune diseases have exploded in prevalence over the past fifty years. Current estimates suggest that approximately 50 million Americans suffer from autoimmune conditions - more than heart disease and cancer combined.[119] The American Autoimmune Related Diseases Association recognizes over 100 distinct autoimmune diseases, with evidence suggesting that many more conditions have autoimmune components.[120] From rheumatoid arthritis to multiple sclerosis, from Hashimoto's thyroiditis to lupus, these conditions share a common feature: the immune system attacking the body's own tissues.

This chapter provides an overview of how autoimmune conditions arise from MILA dysfunction - the same terrain collapse that produces metabolic and cardiovascular disease. For readers seeking comprehensive coverage of autoimmune conditions, including detailed protocols for specific diseases, I refer you to Volume Three of this series, Autoimmune Remission, which addresses these conditions in depth. Here, our focus is on understanding how autoimmunity fits within the unified framework of chronic disease.

The Autoimmune Epidemic

The rise of autoimmune disease cannot be explained by genetics. Genes don't change in decades, but autoimmune prevalence has roughly tripled since the 1970s.[3] Something in our environment - or more precisely, something in the interaction between our environment and our immune systems - has fundamentally shifted.

Several patterns characterize this epidemic. First, autoimmune diseases disproportionately affect women, who comprise approximately 80 percent of autoimmune patients.[121] This gender disparity suggests hormonal influences on immune function - influences that may make women's immune systems more reactive and thus more prone to losing self-tolerance.

Second, autoimmune diseases cluster. A person with one autoimmune condition is significantly more likely to develop others.[122] This clustering suggests that autoimmunity is not simply bad luck affecting random organs but a systemic problem with immune regulation that manifests wherever individual vulnerabilities exist.

Third, autoimmune diseases increasingly appear alongside metabolic conditions. Patients with Hashimoto's thyroiditis have elevated rates of diabetes. Patients with rheumatoid arthritis have increased cardiovascular risk. Patients with inflammatory bowel disease have higher rates of metabolic syndrome.[123] These associations are not coincidental - they reflect the common MILA dysfunction that underlies all chronic disease.

How Self-Tolerance Fails

The immune system is trained from birth to recognize self-tissues as friendly. In the thymus, developing T cells are exposed to the body's own proteins. Those that react too strongly to self are eliminated; those that pass this screening are released to patrol the body.[124] This process, called central tolerance, creates an immune system that should ignore self while remaining capable of responding to foreign threats.

But central tolerance is imperfect. Some self-reactive immune cells escape screening and enter circulation. The body maintains additional safeguards - peripheral tolerance mechanisms - to prevent these escaped cells from causing damage.[125] Regulatory T cells suppress self-reactive responses.

Anti-inflammatory signals counterbalance pro-inflammatory activation. Self-reactive cells that encounter their targets without proper co-stimulation become anergic - functionally inactivated.

Autoimmunity develops when these peripheral tolerance mechanisms fail. The self-reactive cells that should remain suppressed become activated. The regulatory cells that should control them become overwhelmed or dysfunctional. The inflammatory responses that should resolve become self-perpetuating. The result is immune attack on the body's own tissues.

The Triggers of Autoimmune Activation

Research has identified several mechanisms by which self-tolerance breaks down. Understanding these mechanisms reveals how MILA dysfunction creates the conditions for autoimmune disease.

Molecular Mimicry

Some infectious agents carry proteins that structurally resemble human proteins. When the immune system mounts a response against the infection, antibodies and immune cells trained to recognize the pathogen may cross-react with the similar-looking self-tissues.[126] The infection resolves, but the autoimmune response continues - the immune system now targeting the body's own proteins that happen to look like the original invader.

Rheumatic fever provides a classic example. Streptococcal bacteria carry proteins that resemble cardiac tissue. Following strep infection, some patients develop immune responses that attack their own hearts, causing lasting damage.[127] Similar mechanisms have been implicated in multiple sclerosis, type 1 diabetes, and numerous other autoimmune conditions.

Intestinal Permeability

The intestinal lining serves as a critical barrier between the body's internal environment and the external world of the gut lumen. This barrier must perform a delicate balancing act - allowing nutrients to pass while blocking pathogens, toxins, and undigested food particles.[128] When this barrier becomes compromised - a condition sometimes called "leaky gut" - substances that should remain in the gut escape into the bloodstream.

The immune system encounters these escaped particles and mounts responses against them. If any of these particles resemble self-tissues, molecular mimicry ensues. If the chronic presence of foreign material in the bloodstream overwhelms regulatory mechanisms, generalized immune activation results. [129] Research has implicated intestinal permeability in the development of numerous autoimmune conditions, from celiac disease to type 1 diabetes to rheumatoid arthritis.[130]

Notably, intestinal barrier function depends heavily on factors we've already discussed. Chronic inflammation damages the tight junctions between intestinal cells. Mitochondrial dysfunction in intestinal cells impairs their ability to maintain barrier integrity. Lymphatic congestion in the gut allows inflammatory debris to accumulate.[131] MILA dysfunction creates leaky gut, which drives autoimmunity, which worsens MILA dysfunction - another vicious cycle.

Chronic Inflammation and Bystander Activation

Persistent inflammation creates an environment in which autoimmune activation becomes more likely. Inflammatory cytokines lower the threshold for immune cell activation. Tissue damage exposes self-proteins that are normally hidden from immune surveillance.[132] Regulatory T cells, overwhelmed by constant inflammatory signaling, become exhausted and less effective.

"Bystander activation" occurs when inflammation from one source activates self-reactive immune cells that happen to be nearby. The cells weren't specifically triggered by self-tissue, but the inflammatory environment provided the activation signals that broke their tolerance.[133] This mechanism helps explain why autoimmune flares often follow infections, injuries, or periods of stress - any source of inflammation can provide the activating signal.

Autoimmunity Through the MILA Lens

Understanding autoimmunity through the MILA framework reveals why these conditions have become so prevalent and why conventional treatment so often fails.

Mitochondrial dysfunction contributes to autoimmunity in multiple ways. The Cell Danger Response releases mitochondrial components - DNA fragments, ATP, and other molecules - that the immune system recognizes as danger signals.[43] These signals trigger inflammatory responses that can become self-perpetuating. Additionally, mitochondrial dysfunction in immune cells themselves impairs their ability to properly regulate responses - Tregs require substantial energy to function, and energy deficit compromises their regulatory capacity.[134]

Immune dysregulation is, by definition, the core problem in autoimmunity. But this dysregulation doesn't occur in isolation - it reflects upstream dysfunction in the systems that should maintain immune balance. Inadequate Treg function, failure of inflammation resolution, and chronic immune activation all trace back to the broader MILA collapse that affects every aspect of physiology.[48]

Lymphatic impairment prevents clearance of the immune complexes and inflammatory debris that accumulate during autoimmune responses. This accumulation perpetuates inflammation and tissue damage.[8] The lymphatic system also transports antigens to lymph nodes for immune processing -

dysfunction in this transport may contribute to inappropriate immune activation against self-antigens.

Why Immunosuppression Is Not the Answer

Conventional treatment for autoimmune disease focuses on suppressing the immune response - reducing the attack on self-tissues by reducing immune activity overall. Medications range from corticosteroids to disease-modifying anti-rheumatic drugs (DMARDs) to biologics that target specific immune pathways.[135]

These medications can provide symptomatic relief and slow disease progression. They are sometimes necessary and even life-saving in severe disease. But they do not address why the immune system lost tolerance in the first place. They suppress symptoms while the underlying dysfunction continues. And they create new problems by impairing the immune functions that the body needs for defense against infection and cancer surveillance.

Patients on immunosuppressive therapy have increased rates of serious infections.[33] They have elevated cancer risk, particularly for lymphomas and skin cancers.[136] They often require escalating medication doses as their diseases progress despite treatment. The medications manage symptoms while the terrain dysfunction that drove autoimmunity worsens - in part because immunosuppression itself impairs the very healing processes that might restore balance.

The alternative approach - addressing the terrain dysfunction that allowed autoimmunity to develop - offers something immunosuppression cannot: the possibility of restored immune regulation rather than merely suppressed immune activity. When the triggers are removed, when the intestinal barrier heals, when inflammation resolves, when mitochondrial function normalizes - the immune system often regains its ability to distinguish self from non-self. This is not suppression. This is restoration.

The Path to Autoimmune Remission

Autoimmune remission - not just symptom control, but actual restoration of normal immune regulation - is possible for many patients. Studies have documented remission rates of 30 to 50 percent or higher with comprehensive lifestyle and dietary interventions.[137] These results exceed what immunosuppressive medications typically achieve, without the side effects of chronic immune suppression.

The approach follows the same principles we've discussed throughout this book. Remove the triggers that are driving immune activation - inflammatory foods, environmental toxins, chronic infections. Heal the intestinal barrier that may be allowing inappropriate immune stimulation. Resolve the chronic inflammation that is overwhelming regulatory mechanisms. Restore mitochondrial function so that immune cells have the energy they need to regulate properly. Support lymphatic drainage so that immune debris can clear.

The R.E.S.T.O.R.E. MILA protocol addresses each of these factors in sequence. For readers with autoimmune conditions, I strongly recommend Volume Three of this series, which provides detailed protocols tailored to specific autoimmune diseases. The principles are consistent with everything presented in this book - but the specifics matter when addressing conditions as complex as autoimmunity.

Autoimmune conditions demonstrate how immune dysregulation - one pillar of MILA - can become the dominant feature of chronic disease. But immune dysfunction affects more than just autoimmunity. In the next chapter, we will explore neurological conditions, where immune activation in the brain combines with mitochondrial failure and impaired waste clearance to produce cognitive decline, neurodegeneration, and the epidemic of brain-related disorders that increasingly characterizes modern life.

• Key Takeaways

- Autoimmune diseases have tripled in prevalence over the past fifty years, now affecting approximately 50 million Americans - an epidemic that cannot be explained by genetics and must reflect environmental and lifestyle changes affecting immune regulation.

- Autoimmunity develops when peripheral tolerance mechanisms fail, allowing self-reactive immune cells to become activated and attack the body's own tissues through processes including molecular mimicry, intestinal permeability, and chronic inflammatory bystander activation.

- Intestinal barrier dysfunction - leaky gut - plays a critical role in autoimmune development by allowing foreign particles into the bloodstream where they can trigger immune responses that cross-react with self-tissues.

- MILA dysfunction underlies autoimmunity just as it underlies metabolic and cardiovascular disease, with mitochondrial stress releasing danger signals, immune dysregulation losing self-tolerance, and lymphatic impairment preventing clearance of inflammatory debris.

- Conventional immunosuppressive treatment manages symptoms while allowing terrain dysfunction to continue, creating increased risk of infection and cancer while failing to restore actual immune regulation.

- Autoimmune remission is achievable through comprehensive approaches that address underlying triggers and restore terrain function, with studies documenting remission rates of 30 to 50 percent or higher - outcomes that immunosuppression cannot match.

Chapter 6

Neurological Conditions: Brain Fog, Cognitive Decline, and Beyond

Evelyn had always been sharp. At fifty-eight, this former software engineer had spent her career solving complex problems, managing intricate projects, leading teams through technical challenges that would have overwhelmed most people. Her mind had been her greatest asset - quick, precise, reliable. Until it wasn't.

"It started with little things," she told me, her voice carrying the quiet fear of someone watching their identity slip away. "Forgetting where I put my keys. Losing track of what I was saying mid-sentence. Walking into a room and having no idea why I was there. I told myself it was normal aging. Everyone forgets things, right?"

She paused, gathering herself. "But then it got worse. I couldn't follow conversations the way I used to. Technical discussions that would have been easy for me became impossible to track. I started making mistakes at work - stupid mistakes, things I would never have done before. My doctor ran some tests and said my cognition was 'declining faster than expected for my age.' He mentioned early-onset dementia as a possibility. Said we should 'monitor it.'"

Evelyn's eyes met mine. "Monitor it. Watch my brain disappear and do nothing about it. That's what he was offering me. I refuse to accept that."

Evelyn's refusal to accept passive decline was the first step toward her recovery. What her doctor hadn't told her - what conventional neurology rarely acknowledges - is that cognitive decline is not an inevitable consequence of aging. It is a consequence of brain terrain dysfunction - the same MILA collapse that produces every other chronic disease we've discussed. And like those other conditions, it can often be reversed when the underlying dysfunction is addressed.

The Brain Under Siege

Neurological conditions have reached epidemic proportions. Alzheimer's disease alone affects nearly seven million Americans, with projections suggesting this will reach thirteen million by 2050.[5] Parkinson's disease affects over one million Americans and is increasing in prevalence.[138] Multiple sclerosis, once rare, now affects nearly one million people in the United States.[139] And these diagnosed conditions represent only the tip of the iceberg.

Beneath the formal diagnoses lies a vast population experiencing what might be called "subclinical" brain dysfunction - the brain fog, memory problems, concentration difficulties, and processing slowdowns that affect millions who don't yet meet criteria for neurological disease.[140] These symptoms are often dismissed as stress, aging, or simply "normal." They are not normal. They are early warning signs of brain terrain dysfunction that, left unaddressed, may progress to diagnosable neurological disease.

The conventional approach to neurological disease mirrors the approach to other chronic conditions - symptom management without addressing root causes. Alzheimer's medications provide modest symptomatic improvement while doing nothing to halt disease progression. Parkinson's medications replace depleted neurotransmitters while the neurodegeneration continues. Patients are told their conditions are progressive and incurable, that the best they can hope for is slowing the decline. This narrative is incomplete at best and harmful at worst.

The Brain's Energy Crisis

The brain is the most energy-demanding organ in the body. Comprising only two percent of body weight, it consumes approximately twenty percent of the body's oxygen and glucose. [28] Neurons fire constantly, maintaining electrochemical gradients, synthesizing neurotransmitters, processing information at speeds that dwarf any computer. This relentless activity requires enormous ATP production - production that depends entirely on mitochondrial function.

When mitochondrial function declines, the brain is among the first organs to suffer. Unlike muscles, which can switch to less efficient glycolysis when mitochondria fail, neurons have limited metabolic flexibility.[180] They require constant ATP to maintain the ion gradients that make neural signaling possible. Even brief energy deficits can impair cognition. Chronic energy deficits lead to progressive dysfunction and eventually to neuronal death.

Research has consistently documented mitochondrial dysfunction in neurodegenerative diseases. Alzheimer's patients show reduced mitochondrial enzyme activity in affected brain regions.[141] Parkinson's disease involves specific defects in mitochondrial complex I.[143] Multiple sclerosis is associated with mitochondrial damage in both neurons and supporting glial cells.[144] The pattern is consistent: neurological disease correlates with brain energy failure.

This understanding has led some researchers to reconceptualize Alzheimer's disease as "Type 3 diabetes" - a metabolic disorder of the brain in which neurons become insulin resistant and cannot properly utilize glucose for energy.[145] The amyloid plaques and tau tangles that characterize Alzheimer's may be consequences of this metabolic failure rather than primary causes - downstream effects of neurons struggling to survive in an energy-depleted environment.

The Fire in the Brain: Neuroinflammation

The brain was long considered "immune privileged" - protected from the inflammatory processes that affect the rest of the body. We now know this view is incorrect. The brain has its own immune system, centered on glial cells called microglia, and this system can become chronically activated just like peripheral immunity.[146]

Neuroinflammation - chronic immune activation in the brain - is now recognized as a key driver of neurological disease. Activated microglia release inflammatory cytokines that damage neurons. They produce reactive oxygen species that cause oxidative stress. They prune synaptic connections more aggressively than normal, disrupting neural networks.[147] In Alzheimer's disease, activated microglia cluster around amyloid plaques, potentially driving disease progression as much as the plaques themselves.[148]

What triggers neuroinflammation? The same factors that trigger inflammation elsewhere: mitochondrial dysfunction releasing danger signals, systemic inflammation crossing the blood-brain barrier, infections (both acute and chronic), toxin exposure, and metabolic dysfunction.[149] The brain is not isolated from the body. Inflammation anywhere can become inflammation everywhere, including the brain.

This connection between systemic inflammation and brain inflammation helps explain the observed associations between chronic diseases and dementia risk. Patients with diabetes have significantly elevated Alzheimer's risk.[150] Patients with cardiovascular disease have increased cognitive decline.[151] Patients with autoimmune conditions have higher rates of neurological symptoms.[152] These associations are not coincidental - they reflect the common MILA dysfunction that underlies all chronic disease, now manifesting in the brain.

The Glymphatic System: Washing the Brain

Perhaps the most important neuroscience discovery of the past two decades has been the glymphatic system - the brain's waste clearance network that was only identified in 2012.[23] This discovery revolutionized our understanding of brain health and disease.

The glymphatic system uses cerebrospinal fluid to flush metabolic waste from brain tissue. This fluid flows through channels formed by astrocytes - star-shaped glial cells that wrap around blood vessels. As it flows, it carries away the debris of neural metabolism: damaged proteins, metabolic byproducts, and notably, the amyloid-beta and tau proteins that accumulate in Alzheimer's disease.[55]

The critical finding: glymphatic clearance occurs primarily during deep sleep. During wakefulness, brain cells are tightly packed together, leaving little space for fluid flow. During deep sleep, these cells shrink by approximately sixty percent, opening channels through which cerebrospinal fluid can surge.[29] A single night of sleep deprivation significantly reduces amyloid-beta clearance.[153] Chronic sleep deprivation allows waste to accumulate day after day, potentially contributing to long-term neurodegeneration.

This discovery explains the well-documented association between sleep disorders and dementia risk. People with chronic insomnia have elevated Alzheimer's risk.[154] Sleep apnea - which fragments sleep and reduces time in deep stages - is strongly associated with cognitive decline.[155] Sleep is not merely rest for the brain. It is active maintenance - the time when accumulated waste is cleared and the neural environment is restored.

Glymphatic function also depends on factors beyond sleep. Adequate hydration maintains the fluid pressure needed for clearance. Body position affects flow - side sleeping appears more effective than back sleeping. Exercise enhances glymphatic function through mechanisms not yet fully understood. And notably, inflammation impairs glymphatic flow, creating another connection between MILA dysfunction and brain health.

The Brain Through the MILA Lens

Understanding neurological conditions through the MILA framework integrates these various mechanisms into a coherent picture - and reveals why conventional approaches fail while suggesting what might actually work.

Mitochondrial dysfunction deprives neurons of the ATP they need to function. The brain enters an energy crisis, unable to maintain normal activity. Neurons that cannot generate sufficient ATP become dysfunctional and eventually die. The Cell Danger Response, triggered by mitochondrial stress, releases signals that activate neuroinflammation.[6]

Immune dysregulation manifests as chronic microglial activation. The brain's immune cells, receiving persistent danger signals, remain in a state of chronic inflammation. They release cytokines that damage neurons, prune synapses excessively, and create an environment hostile to normal brain function.[156]

Lymphatic impairment - specifically glymphatic dysfunction - prevents clearance of the metabolic waste and inflammatory debris accumulating in brain tissue. Proteins aggregate. Inflammation persists. The neural environment becomes progressively more toxic.[157]

These three dysfunctions feed each other in the same vicious cycle we have seen in other organs. Mitochondrial failure triggers inflammation. Inflammation impairs glymphatic flow. Poor clearance allows waste to accumulate, further stressing mitochondria. The spiral continues until clinical disease manifests

- as brain fog, as cognitive decline, eventually as diagnosable neurodegeneration.

Reversing Cognitive Decline

The conventional narrative holds that neurological decline is irreversible - that lost neurons cannot be replaced and lost function cannot be restored. This narrative is increasingly challenged by research demonstrating that cognitive improvement is possible, even in patients with early-stage dementia.[158]

Dr. Dale Bredesen's research on "metabolic enhancement for neurodegeneration" has documented cognitive improvement in Alzheimer's patients using a comprehensive protocol addressing multiple factors - diet, exercise, sleep, stress, toxin exposure, and targeted supplementation.[159] Patients who had been declining showed measurable improvement in cognitive testing. Some returned to work after having been forced to quit due to cognitive impairment. The key was addressing multiple mechanisms simultaneously rather than targeting any single factor.

This approach aligns perfectly with the MILA framework and the R.E.S.T.O.R.E. MILA protocol. Cognitive decline doesn't have a single cause, so it can't be fixed with a single intervention. But when mitochondrial function is restored, when neuroinflammation is calmed, when glymphatic clearance is optimized, when the brain terrain is restored - improvement becomes possible. Not guaranteed, not universal, but possible in ways that conventional neurology does not acknowledge.

Evelyn's Return

Evelyn's assessment revealed what I had expected: markers of systemic inflammation, signs of metabolic dysfunction, and a sleep study showing fragmented sleep with minimal time in the deep stages critical for glymphatic clearance. Her brain wasn't failing at random - it was failing for specific, identifiable, addressable reasons.

"Your brain isn't broken," I told her. "It's starving and drowning at the same time - starving for energy because your mitochondria aren't functioning optimally and drowning in waste because you're not getting the deep sleep needed to clear it. We can address both of these."

The protocol focused first on sleep - optimizing sleep hygiene, addressing the factors disrupting her sleep architecture, and in her case, treating previously undiagnosed mild sleep apnea. Within three weeks, Evelyn reported waking more refreshed than she had in years.

Anti-inflammatory nutrition came next, removing the dietary factors contributing to systemic and neuroinflammation. Then mitochondrial support - CoQ10, B vitamins, and other nutrients that support ATP production. Movement to stimulate both mitochondrial biogenesis and glymphatic flow. Stress reduction to lower the cortisol that was impairing both sleep and cognitive function.

The changes came gradually but unmistakably. By month two, Evelyn noticed she was losing her keys less often. By month three, she could follow technical discussions again. By month six, her cognitive testing showed improvement that her neurologist described as "unexpected" - a revealing word choice that showed how thoroughly conventional medicine has accepted decline as inevitable.

"I got my brain back," she told me at her nine-month follow-up. "Not just holding steady - actually better than when I first came to see you. I'm doing things I had stopped doing because I couldn't handle them cognitively. My doctor says he's never seen anything like it. I told him maybe he should start looking."

Evelyn's recovery was not miraculous. It was biological. When the obstacles to brain function were removed, when the conditions for neural health were restored, her brain did what brains are designed to do - it healed.

The brain, like every other organ, depends on MILA function for health. When mitochondria fail, when inflammation rages, when waste clearance stalls, neurological disease follows. But one condition sits at the intersection of all chronic disease, affecting virtually every patient with MILA dysfunction: chronic fatigue. In the next chapter, we will explore chronic fatigue syndrome and fibromyalgia, revealing how these conditions represent the Cell Danger Response in its purest form - and why understanding them illuminates the path to recovery from all chronic disease.

Key Takeaways

- Neurological conditions from brain fog to dementia have reached epidemic proportions, with Alzheimer's disease alone projected to affect thirteen million Americans by 2050, yet conventional medicine offers only symptom management rather than addressing root causes.

- The brain consumes twenty percent of the body's energy while comprising only two percent of body weight, making it exquisitely sensitive to mitochondrial dysfunction - which has been documented in Alzheimer's, Parkinson's, multiple sclerosis, and virtually every neurodegenerative condition.

- Neuroinflammation - chronic immune activation in the brain mediated by microglia - is now recognized as a key driver of neurological disease, triggered by the same factors that cause inflammation elsewhere: mitochondrial dysfunction, systemic inflammation, infections, and toxin exposure.

- The glymphatic system clears metabolic waste from the brain primarily during deep sleep, making sleep optimization essential for brain health and explaining the strong association between sleep disorders and dementia risk.

- MILA dysfunction in the brain follows the same pattern as elsewhere: mitochondrial failure triggers neuroinflammation, inflammation impairs glymphatic clearance, poor clearance allows waste accumulation that further stresses mitochondria - a vicious cycle leading to progressive cognitive decline.

- Research has demonstrated that cognitive improvement is possible even in early-stage dementia when multiple factors are addressed simultaneously - restoring mitochondrial function, calming neuroinflammation, and optimizing glymphatic clearance through sleep, nutrition, and lifestyle interventions.

Chapter 7

Chronic Fatigue and Fibromyalgia: The Cell Danger Response

Helen used to run marathons. At forty-four, this emergency room nurse had completed twelve of them, rising before dawn to train while managing a demanding career and raising two teenagers. She had energy to spare. Then came the flu that changed everything.

"It was just a bad flu," she told me, her voice flat with exhaustion. "Everyone gets the flu. But I never recovered. Three years later, I'm still waiting to feel like myself again."

Helen's symptoms were devastating in their totality. Crushing fatigue that made getting out of bed feel like climbing a mountain. Muscle pain was so severe that a hug from her children made her wince. Brain fog was so thick that she had to quit the job she had loved for fifteen years because she couldn't trust herself to make critical decisions. Sleep that never refreshed, no matter how many hours she spent in bed. Crashes after any exertion that would leave her bedridden for days.

"I've seen eleven doctors," she continued. "They've run every test imaginable. Everything comes back normal. One of them actually told me it was all in my head - that I should see a psychiatrist. As if I'm imagining that I can't walk to my mailbox without needing to rest afterward."

Helen had been diagnosed with chronic fatigue syndrome - a label that describes her symptoms without explaining them. She had also been told she had fibromyalgia, based on her widespread pain. What no one had explained was why her body had seemingly shut down, why it refused to recover, and whether recovery was even possible. Conventional medicine had nothing to offer but symptom management - pain medications, sleep aids, antidepressants - none of which addressed what was actually wrong.

What Helen was experiencing was not mysterious. It was not psychological. It was not imaginary. It was the Cell Danger Response - the most fundamental survival mechanism in human biology - stuck in the "on" position. And understanding this transforms both how we view these conditions and how we treat them.

The Invisible Epidemic

Chronic fatigue syndrome (CFS), also known as myalgic encephalomyelitis (ME), affects an estimated 2.5 million Americans.[160] Fibromyalgia affects approximately 4 million more.[161] Many patients have both conditions, which overlap substantially in symptoms and likely share underlying mechanisms. These are not rare diseases - they are epidemic conditions that have been largely ignored by mainstream medicine.

The economic and personal costs are staggering. CFS alone costs the US economy approximately 17 to 24 billion dollars annually in lost productivity and medical expenses.[162] More than one-quarter of CFS patients are bedbound or housebound at some point in their illness.[163] Quality of life scores for CFS patients are lower than for patients with multiple sclerosis, heart failure, or cancer undergoing chemotherapy.[164] These are seriously ill people whose suffering is routinely dismissed.

The dismissal stems partly from the invisibility of these conditions. Patients look normal. Standard lab tests come back normal. Imaging studies show no obvious pathology. Without a visible lesion or abnormal blood marker to point to, many physicians conclude that the problem must be psychological - an assumption that has caused immense harm and delayed effective treatment for millions.

But the tests were looking for the wrong things. These patients don't have organ damage visible on imaging. They have cellular energy failure that requires specialized testing to detect. Their mitochondria are not producing adequate ATP. Their cells are stuck in survival mode. Standard medical testing does not assess mitochondrial function - so it misses the core problem entirely.[20]

The Cell Danger Response: Survival Mode Gone Chronic

We introduced the Cell Danger Response in Chapter 1, but its role in chronic fatigue and fibromyalgia is so central that it warrants deeper exploration. The CDR, as described by Dr. Robert Naviaux, is the evolutionary conserved metabolic response that cells mount when they detect danger - whether from infection, toxin exposure, physical trauma, or severe stress. [6]

The CDR is not a malfunction. It is an intelligent, coordinated survival program that has protected life for billions of years. When mitochondria sense danger, they initiate a cascade of changes designed to help the cell survive an acute threat. These changes include shifting from efficient aerobic metabolism to less efficient but faster glycolysis, releasing danger signals to alert neighboring cells and the immune system, reducing responsiveness to normal hormonal signals, and closing communication channels with other cells.

In acute illness, this response is lifesaving. It prioritizes immediate survival over normal function. Energy production decreases, but enough is maintained to keep the cell alive. Inflammation activates to fight the threat. The body hunkers down, riding out the storm until the danger passes.

The problem arises when the CDR doesn't turn off. The response was designed for temporary activation - days to weeks during acute illness. When it persists for months or years, it creates the syndrome we call chronic fatigue.[165] The body remains in survival mode indefinitely, energy production chronically suppressed, inflammation chronically elevated, normal function chronically impaired.

Research has documented this phenomenon in CFS patients. Metabolomic studies reveal a characteristic pattern of hypometabolism - cellular energy production running far below normal.[166] The metabolic signature resembles hibernation or dauer (a survival state in certain organisms) more than normal human physiology.[167] Cells are deliberately conserving resources, operating at minimum capacity, waiting for an "all clear" signal that never comes.

Why the Cell Danger Response Gets Stuck

If the CDR is designed to be temporary, why does it become chronic? Several factors can prevent the body from completing the healing cycle and returning to normal function.

Persistent Triggers

The most obvious reason the CDR stays activated is that the danger hasn't actually passed. Chronic infections - whether viral, bacterial, or parasitic - can smolder for years, continuously triggering the danger response.[168] Environmental toxins accumulating in tissues maintain the alert state. Chronic inflammatory foods keep the immune system activated. Ongoing psychological stress keeps stress hormones elevated. As long as the body perceives danger, it maintains the survival response.

Insufficient Resources for Recovery

The transition from CDR back to normal metabolism requires energy and specific nutrients. If the body lacks the resources needed to exit survival mode, it remains stuck there.[169] This creates a cruel irony: the hypometabolic state reduces the very energy production needed to escape it. The CDR becomes self-perpetuating, trapping patients in a low-energy state they cannot climb out of without support.

Failed Inflammation Resolution

Inflammation is supposed to resolve once threats are eliminated. The body produces specialized pro-resolving mediators (SPMs) that actively terminate inflammatory responses and initiate healing.[170] But SPM production requires adequate omega-3 fatty acids and properly functioning enzymatic pathways. When these are deficient - as they commonly are in modern Western diets - inflammation cannot properly resolve. It becomes chronic, continuously triggering the CDR.

Impaired Waste Clearance

Lymphatic congestion prevents clearance of the metabolic waste and inflammatory debris generated during the CDR.[171] This waste accumulates in tissues, creating a toxic environment that continues triggering danger signals. The body cannot recognize that the original threat is gone because the debris from fighting it has not been cleared. Again, the modern sedentary lifestyle is implicated - without movement, lymph does not flow, and waste does not clear.

Fibromyalgia: Pain as Part of the Pattern

Fibromyalgia is characterized by widespread musculoskeletal pain, often described as a constant deep ache affecting multiple body regions. For years, the condition was considered psychosomatic because no obvious tissue damage could be found to explain the pain. We now understand that the pain is real - it is just not coming from where conventional medicine was looking.[172]

Research has revealed that fibromyalgia involves central sensitization - the nervous system becomes hypersensitive, amplifying pain signals and interpreting normal stimuli as painful.[173] This explains why fibromyalgia patients experience allodynia (pain from normally non-painful stimuli) and hyperalgesia (excessive pain from mildly painful stimuli). The problem isn't in the muscles themselves - it's in how the nervous system processes signals from those muscles.

Central sensitization fits perfectly into the MILA framework. Neuroinflammation - the same microglial activation we discussed in neurological disease - alters pain processing in the central nervous system.[174] Mitochondrial dysfunction in neurons impairs their ability to properly regulate pain signals. And notably, the CDR includes alterations in pain pathways as part of its survival response - heightened pain sensitivity may have evolved to promote protective behavior during recovery from injury or illness.

This understanding explains why chronic fatigue and fibromyalgia so often occur together. They are not separate diseases that happen to coincide - they are different manifestations of the same underlying process. The CDR produces both the energy deficit of chronic fatigue and the pain amplification of fibromyalgia. Treating them as separate conditions requiring separate approaches misses the unified cause.

The Complete MILA Picture

Chronic fatigue syndrome (CFS) and fibromyalgia represent MILA dysfunction in its most complete form - all three pillars failing simultaneously, with the CDR at the center of the collapse.

Mitochondrial dysfunction is the defining feature. Energy production is severely impaired, running at a fraction of normal capacity.[175] This is not laziness or deconditioning - it's cellular energy failure documented by metabolomic testing. Patients don't lack motivation; they lack ATP.

Immune dysregulation manifests as chronic low-grade inflammation, altered cytokine profiles, and impaired pathogen defense.[176] Many CFS patients report that their illness began with an infection - a viral illness, like Helen's flu, that they never recovered from. The immune system mounted a response but could not properly resolve it. Years later, inflammatory markers remain elevated while actual immune function against new threats is impaired.

Lymphatic impairment prevents clearance of the inflammatory debris and metabolic waste accumulating from chronic CDR activation.[177] Patients often report feeling "toxic" - a subjective experience that reflects the objective reality of waste accumulation in tissues. The characteristic worsening with exertion (post-exertional malaise) may partly reflect increased metabolic waste production that the impaired lymphatic system cannot handle.

These dysfunctions reinforce each other in the familiar vicious cycle. Mitochondrial failure triggers inflammation. Inflammation impairs lymphatic flow. Lymphatic congestion allows waste to accumulate. Accumulated waste further stresses mitochondria. Each attempt the body makes to exit the CDR is thwarted by the downstream consequences of the CDR itself.

Breaking the Cycle: The Path to Recovery

Recovery from chronic fatigue and fibromyalgia is possible - but it requires understanding that these conditions cannot be pushed through. The standard advice to "exercise more" is not merely unhelpful; it can be actively harmful. Exercise increases metabolic demand when the system is already unable to meet normal demand. It generates waste when the lymphatic system is already struggling to clear existing waste. It can trigger prolonged crashes that set recovery back by weeks or months.

The approach must be different - supporting the body's exit from the CDR rather than demanding function it cannot provide. This requires addressing all factors preventing recovery: removing persistent triggers, providing resources for metabolic restoration, supporting inflammation resolution, and optimizing waste clearance.[178]

The R.E.S.T.O.R.E. MILA protocol is specifically designed for this purpose. Its sequence reflects the biological requirements for exiting the CDR. Drainage is addressed first because waste must be able to clear as metabolism increases. Immune regulation comes next because inflammation must resolve for the CDR to lift. Only then is mitochondrial support introduced - once the system is prepared to handle increased energy production.

Pacing - carefully managing activity to stay within available energy limits - is essential during recovery. The goal is to gradually expand capacity rather than repeatedly exceed it. Small improvements build on each other. Energy gradually increases. Function slowly returns. The timeline is months to years, not weeks - but the direction is toward health rather than continued decline.

Helen's Recovery

Helen's assessment confirmed what her symptoms suggested: profound mitochondrial dysfunction, elevated inflammatory markers, and signs of lymphatic congestion. Her body was locked in survival mode, running on minimal energy, unable to exit the CDR that had been triggered three years earlier by a flu virus.

"Your cells went into crisis mode when you got sick," I explained. "That's normal - it's how the body protects itself during acute illness. But something prevented you from coming out of that mode. You've been running on emergency power for three years. No wonder you're exhausted."

The first priority was lymphatic drainage - gentle, passive approaches that wouldn't trigger the crashes that had plagued Helen's previous attempts to improve. Dry brushing. Gentle rebounding. Careful attention to hydration. Within weeks, Helen reported feeling slightly "less toxic" - a subjective improvement that preceded any measurable change.

Anti-inflammatory nutrition came next, removing the dietary factors that were perpetuating her immune activation. Helen had been eating what she thought was a healthy diet, but it included several foods that were triggering inflammatory responses in her system. Removing them reduced one more burden her overwhelmed system was carrying.

Only after three months of drainage and inflammation work did we introduce mitochondrial support - CoQ10, B vitamins, magnesium, and other nutrients that support ATP production. Earlier supplementation would have pushed for energy production the system was not ready to handle. Now, with drainage open and inflammation reduced, her cells could begin to increase their energy output safely.

Progress was slow but steady. By month four, Helen noticed she could do slightly more without crashing. By month six, she was able to take short walks. By month nine, she was walking a mile most days - an accomplishment that would have been unthinkable a year earlier. By month twelve, she was considering returning to work part-time.

"I'm not running marathons again," she told me at her one-year follow-up. "I may never run another marathon. But I have a life again. I can be present for my kids. I can think clearly. I can do things that matter to me. After three years of being told nothing could help me, that feels like a miracle."

It wasn't a miracle. It was biology. Helen's body had been stuck in a survival state, unable to exit on its own. Once the obstacles were removed and the resources for recovery were provided, her system did what it had been trying to do all along - it healed.

Chronic fatigue and fibromyalgia represent MILA dysfunction in its clearest form - the Cell Danger Response visible as a coherent pattern rather than masked as organ-specific disease. Understanding these conditions illuminates the entire spectrum of chronic illness. But understanding alone doesn't heal. The chapters that follow will provide specific protocols for restoration - beginning with the assessment process that reveals each individual's unique pattern of dysfunction and guides the path back to health.

Key Takeaways

- Chronic fatigue syndrome and fibromyalgia affect millions of Americans yet remain poorly understood by conventional medicine, which often dismisses these conditions as psychological when standard tests fail to reveal obvious pathology.

- The Cell Danger Response - the evolutionarily conserved survival program that cells activate during acute threats - becomes chronic in these conditions, leaving the body stuck in a hypometabolic survival state that produces the characteristic symptoms of exhaustion and pain.

- The CDR persists because of factors including ongoing triggers such as chronic infection or toxin exposure, insufficient resources for metabolic recovery, failed inflammation resolution, and impaired lymphatic clearance of metabolic waste.

- Fibromyalgia's widespread pain results from central sensitization - neuroinflammation-driven hypersensitivity in pain processing pathways - which is part of the same CDR pattern that produces chronic fatigue, explaining why these conditions so often occur together.
- Standard advice to exercise more can be actively harmful in these conditions, as increased metabolic demand exceeds available energy capacity and generates waste the lymphatic system cannot clear, potentially triggering prolonged crashes.
- Recovery requires supporting the body's exit from the CDR through careful sequencing - addressing drainage before increasing metabolism, resolving inflammation before stimulating mitochondria - combined with pacing that respects current energy limits while gradually expanding capacity.

Chapter 8

The Three Laws of Healing: Sequence, Synergy, and Patience

Before we explore the specific steps of the R.E.S.T.O.R.E. MILA protocol, we must understand the principles that make it work. These principles explain why so many well-intentioned treatment approaches fail - and why proper sequencing succeeds where random intervention does not. They are not arbitrary rules but reflections of biological reality, of how the body actually heals when given the opportunity.

I call these the Three Laws of Healing: Sequence, Synergy, and Patience. Violate any one of them, and recovery stalls or fails. Honor all three, and the body's remarkable capacity for restoration becomes available.

The First Law: Sequence

The order in which you address dysfunction matters as much as what you address. This seems obvious once stated, yet it is violated constantly in both conventional and functional medicine. Practitioners identify problems and immediately begin treating them - without considering whether the body is prepared to respond to that treatment.

Consider a simple analogy. Imagine a house that has been damaged by a flood. The basement is full of water. The walls are soaked. Mold is growing. The electrical system has been compromised. A well-meaning but poorly sequenced approach might start by repainting the walls - after all, they look terrible. But paint applied to wet walls will peel. Worse, it will trap moisture inside, accelerating mold growth. The correct sequence is clear: pump out the water first, dry the structure, address the mold, repair the electrical system, and only then refinish the surfaces.

The body follows similar logic. You cannot effectively support mitochondrial energy production while the lymphatic system is congested with waste - the increased metabolic activity will generate more waste than can be cleared, triggering inflammation and worsening the condition. You cannot successfully calm inflammation while chronic infections persist - the immune system will continue responding to the ongoing threat regardless of anti-inflammatory interventions. You cannot restore normal hormone function while the liver is overwhelmed with toxins - the liver produces cholesterol and other precursors essential for hormone synthesis, metabolizes and clears used hormones from circulation, and converts thyroid hormone T4 to active T3. A compromised liver disrupts this entire hormonal ecosystem.

This principle of biological sequencing is not new. The concept of "drainage before detoxification" has been recognized in natural medicine for over a century.[179] What the MILA framework adds is understanding of why this sequence matters at the cellular and systemic level - and extension of the principle to encompass the full restoration process.

The R.E.S.T.O.R.E. MILA protocol embodies proper sequencing in its very structure. Each letter represents a phase that must be substantially completed before the next phase can be fully effective. The sequence reflects biological requirements, not arbitrary preference.

The R.E.S.T.O.R.E. Sequence Explained

R - Reveal: Before any intervention can occur, you must understand what you are dealing with. This phase uses comprehensive assessment and baseline testing to reveal exactly what is happening in your body - which systems are most dysfunctional, what triggers are present, and what obstacles must be addressed. You cannot fix a problem you haven't identified.

E - Eliminate: With your baseline established, elimination begins. This means stopping the influx of toxins, increasing lymphatic flow, and opening drainage pathways. You cannot detoxify if your drainage is blocked - toxins released from tissues have nowhere to go and simply recirculate. This phase also eliminates inflammatory foods and environmental exposures that perpetuate dysfunction.

S - Strengthen: With drainage open and toxic burden reducing, the immune system can be strengthened and regulated. This phase addresses immune balance and infection control - supporting the body's ability to manage chronic infections while preventing excessive inflammatory responses. Immune regulation must precede mitochondrial stimulation.

T - Turbocharge: Now the body is ready for mitochondrial support. This phase turbocharges cellular energy production through targeted supplementation supporting mitochondrial function, methylation pathways, and ATP generation. Earlier mitochondrial stimulation often backfires; with proper preparation, it becomes effective and well-tolerated.

O - Optimize: With energy restored, optimization becomes possible. This phase focuses on circadian rhythm restoration, glymphatic system function, and mood stabilization. These systems require adequate cellular energy to function properly - which is why this phase follows rather than precedes mitochondrial support.

R - Repair: The second R phase targets individual problem areas that remain after the foundational phases. This is where personalized intervention addresses specific tissues, organs, or systems that need additional support based on your unique presentation and remaining symptoms.

E - Everlasting: The final phase establishes maintenance for life. This is where the focus shifts from active healing to sustained wellness - the lifestyle practices and minimal supplementation that maintain restored health indefinitely. The goal is not dependency on protocols but freedom from them.

Why Random Approaches Fail

Understanding proper sequence illuminates why so many treatment approaches produce disappointing results. Patients try intervention after intervention, sometimes experiencing temporary improvement, often experiencing nothing, occasionally getting worse. The interventions may be individually sound - the problem is their timing.

Consider a common scenario. A patient with chronic fatigue reads about the benefits of CoQ10 for mitochondrial function.[180] The research is legitimate - CoQ10 does support mitochondrial energy production. The patient begins taking it and initially feels slightly better. But within weeks, the improvement plateaus, or reverses. The patient concludes that CoQ10 "doesn't work for me" and moves on to the next supplement.

What actually happened? The CoQ10 did support increased mitochondrial activity. But the patient's lymphatic system was congested, unable to clear the increased metabolic waste. Inflammation rose. The immune system activated. The brief improvement was overwhelmed by the consequences of out-of-sequence intervention. The supplement wasn't wrong - the timing was.

This pattern repeats endlessly. Patients accumulate collections of supplements they've tried and abandoned, practitioners they've seen and left, protocols they've started and stopped. Each intervention addressed something real. None addressed the foundation required to make it work.

Functional medicine, despite its systems-based philosophy, often falls into this trap. A practitioner identifies mitochondrial dysfunction and immediately begins mitochondrial support. Another identifies gut dysbiosis and immediately begins aggressive gut protocols. A third identifies heavy metal burden and immediately begins chelation. Each is treating real problems. None is respecting the sequence required for those treatments to succeed.

The Second Law: Synergy

The three pillars of MILA do not function independently. They are deeply interconnected, each affecting and affected by the others. Effective treatment must address all three - not necessarily simultaneously, but comprehensively within the overall protocol.

We've seen these connections throughout this book. Mitochondrial dysfunction triggers immune activation through the Cell Danger Response.[6] Immune dysregulation produces inflammation that impairs mitochondrial function.[50] Lymphatic congestion allows inflammatory debris to accumulate, perpetuating both mitochondrial stress and immune activation.[8] The system is interconnected at every level.

This interconnection means that addressing only one pillar produces limited results. You can support mitochondria all day, but if chronic inflammation is suppressing mitochondrial function, improvement will be modest at best. You can calm inflammation repeatedly, but if the lymphatic system isn't clearing inflammatory debris, it will keep returning. You can optimize lymphatic flow, but if mitochondrial dysfunction keeps generating inflammatory signals, the lymphatic system will remain overwhelmed.

The R.E.S.T.O.R.E. MILA protocol addresses all three pillars in proper sequence. Each phase contributes to multiple aspects of MILA function. Drainage supports lymphatic health while reducing inflammatory burden. Anti-inflammatory approaches calm immune overactivation while reducing mitochondrial stress. Mitochondrial support provides energy for immune function and lymphatic pumping. The pieces work together synergistically, each making the others more effective.

This synergy explains why comprehensive protocols outperform single-target interventions. A study comparing single interventions to multimodal approaches for chronic disease consistently shows superior outcomes for the multimodal approach - not because any individual component is better, but because the components work together in ways that amplify their effects.

The Third Law: Patience

Chronic disease develops over years or decades. It will not resolve in days or weeks. This seems obvious, yet impatience derails more healing journeys than any other factor.

Modern medicine has conditioned us to expect rapid results. Take an antibiotic, feel better in days. Take a pain reliever, feel better in hours. This conditioning creates unrealistic expectations for chronic disease treatment. When improvement doesn't come quickly, patients assume the treatment isn't working and abandon it - often just as it was beginning to produce results. [181]

Biological restoration takes time for good reasons. Cells must be rebuilt. Mitochondria must replicate. Neural pathways must be rewired. The microbiome must be repopulated.

Inflammatory patterns must be extinguished. None of this happens overnight, regardless of how aggressive the intervention is.

Consider mitochondrial biogenesis - the process by which cells produce new mitochondria. This process takes weeks to months, even under optimal conditions.[182] A patient with mitochondrial dysfunction won't feel significantly better until new, healthy mitochondria have been produced and dysfunctional ones have been cleared. No amount of supplementation can accelerate this biological timeline.

Similarly, gut microbiome restoration requires time for beneficial species to establish and outcompete harmful ones.[183] Neural plasticity - the brain's ability to reorganize itself - operates on timescales of months to years.[184] Immune memory must fade before new patterns can be established.[185] These are not optional delays but biological necessities.

Patience also means accepting non-linear progress. Healing rarely proceeds in a straight line. There are good days and bad days, good weeks and difficult weeks. Symptoms may temporarily intensify as the body processes accumulated toxins or old infections reactivate during immune restoration. These fluctuations are normal - often they indicate that healing is occurring, not that treatment is failing.

The healing journey typically follows a pattern: initial stabilization, gradual improvement with fluctuations, increasing stability as improvements consolidate, and eventual establishment of a new baseline substantially better than where the patient started. This pattern unfolds over months to years, not days to weeks. Patients who understand this timeline can persist through difficult periods. Those who expect rapid results often quit before the real improvement begins.

Applying the Three Laws

The Three Laws provide a framework for evaluating any treatment approach. When considering an intervention, ask three questions:

Is the sequence correct? Is my body prepared for this intervention? Have the prerequisite phases been addressed? Am I trying to build before the foundation is laid?

Does it support synergy? Does this intervention work with my overall protocol? Does it address the interconnected nature of MILA dysfunction? Or does it focus narrowly on one aspect while ignoring the others?

Am I being patient? Am I giving this intervention adequate time to work? Am I expecting results faster than biology allows? Am I mistaking normal fluctuations for treatment failure?

These questions can prevent the random, reactive approach to treatment that characterizes so many failed healing attempts. They provide a rational basis for decision-making that respects biological reality rather than fighting against it.

What to Expect in the Chapters Ahead

The chapters that follow will guide you through each phase of the R.E.S.T.O.R.E. MILA protocol in detail. You will learn specific strategies for recognizing and removing obstacles, establishing drainage, soothing inflammation, transforming terrain, optimizing mitochondria, regulating immunity, and sustaining your gains.

For each phase, we will cover the underlying principles, specific interventions, how to assess progress, and when to move forward. The information is designed to be practical and actionable while remaining grounded in the science we've explored throughout this book.

Remember that this is a framework, not a rigid prescription. Every person's situation is unique. The specific interventions that work best will vary based on individual factors - genetic predispositions, specific dysfunctions, resources available, and personal preferences. The protocol provides structure; you and your healthcare provider adapt it to your circumstances.

Finally, remember why proper sequencing matters. The patients whose stories we've shared throughout this book - Margaret, David, Gloria, Raymond, Evelyn, Helen - all followed this sequenced approach. Their recoveries weren't random or lucky. They were the predictable result of addressing dysfunction in the order that biology demands. The same possibility exists for anyone willing to honor the Three Laws of Healing.

With these principles established, we are ready to begin the protocol itself. The next chapter addresses the first phase: Reveal. Before any intervention can succeed, you must understand exactly what is happening in your body - which systems are most dysfunctional, what triggers are present, and what your baseline looks like. Assessment creates the roadmap for everything that follows.

Key Takeaways

- The Three Laws of Healing - Sequence, Synergy, and Patience - provide the framework that makes the R.E.S.T.O.R.E. MILA protocol effective, explaining why random interventions fail while properly ordered approaches succeed.

- Sequence requires that each phase of healing prepares the body for the next, just as draining a flooded basement must precede repainting the walls - you cannot effectively support mitochondria while lymphatic drainage is impaired or calm inflammation while triggers persist.

- The R.E.S.T.O.R.E. sequence reflects biological requirements: Reveal through assessment, Eliminate toxins and open drainage, Strengthen immune regulation, Turbocharge mitochondria, Optimize circadian and glymphatic function, Repair individual problem areas, and Everlasting maintenance for life.

- Synergy recognizes that the three MILA pillars are deeply interconnected, meaning effective treatment must address all three comprehensively - supporting any single pillar while ignoring the others produces limited results.

- Patience accepts that chronic disease developed over years and will not resolve in weeks, with biological processes like mitochondrial biogenesis, microbiome restoration, and immune memory requiring months to years regardless of intervention intensity.

- Healing progress is typically non-linear with good days and difficult days, and temporary symptom intensification may indicate that healing is occurring rather than that treatment is failing.

Chapter 9

R - Reveal: Assessment and Baseline Testing

Before you can fix a problem, you must understand what the problem actually is. This seems obvious, yet the majority of chronic disease treatment occurs without genuine understanding of the underlying dysfunction. Patients receive diagnoses that describe symptoms without explaining causes. They take medications that alter biomarkers without addressing why those markers became abnormal. They try supplement after supplement, hoping something will work, without a map to guide their choices.

The Reveal phase changes this. It creates clarity where confusion existed, replacing guesswork with precision. Before any intervention can succeed, you must know which systems are most dysfunctional, what triggers are perpetuating the problem, and what your baseline looks like so you can measure progress. Assessment creates the roadmap for everything that follows.

Why Assessment Comes First

Consider what happens when someone with chronic fatigue starts taking CoQ10 without proper assessment. The research supporting CoQ10 for mitochondrial function is legitimate.[180] But if that person has severe lymphatic congestion, the increased mitochondrial activity generates more metabolic waste than their drainage system can handle. Symptoms worsen. The patient concludes that CoQ10 doesn't work for them and moves on to the next supplement.

The problem wasn't the supplement - it was the lack of assessment revealing that drainage needed to be addressed first. This pattern repeats endlessly in both conventional and functional medicine. Patients accumulate collections of supplements they've tried and abandoned, practitioners they've seen and left, protocols they've started and stopped. Each intervention addressed something real. None addressed the foundation required to make it work.

The detoxification industry has convinced millions that they can cleanse their way to health, that the solution to feeling toxic is aggressive removal protocols. Bottles of milk thistle, NAC, chlorella, and activated charcoal line the shelves of health food stores, each promising to cleanse your liver or eliminate toxins.[186] But here's what they don't tell you: detoxification is not the first step. Before you can mobilize toxins from tissues, you need functioning drainage pathways to eliminate them. Before you can support liver conjugation, you need to open lymphatic channels to transport toxins to the liver. Before you can bind toxins in the gut, you need proper bowel motility to actually remove them from your body.

The R.E.S.T.O.R.E. MILA protocol begins with Reveal precisely because clarity must precede action. Guessing is expensive - both financially and physiologically. Taking supplements blindly wastes money at best and causes harm at worst.[187] The Reveal phase creates the map that prevents misdirected therapy and allows every subsequent intervention to be precise, targeted, and effective.

What Reveal Actually Means

To reveal is to see clearly what's hidden. In the context of MILA dysfunction, this means identifying the unique combination of mitochondrial stress, immune imbalance, and lymphatic stagnation creating your symptoms. This isn't about collecting data for data's sake - it's about asking the right questions so you can implement the right solutions in the right sequence.

Most conventional medicine operates on a model I call "test-and-treat." Run labs. Find abnormalities. Prescribe medications that force markers back into "normal" ranges.[188] The problem? Normal ranges don't equal optimal function. You can have "normal" TSH with profound hypothyroid symptoms. "Normal" vitamin B12 with severe neurological deficits. "Normal" ferritin with crushing fatigue.[189] The numbers look fine on paper while you feel terrible in reality.

The MILA framework shifts the question from "Are your numbers normal?" to "Is your system functioning?" These are fundamentally different inquiries. The first looks at static snapshots. The second examines dynamic processes - the flow of energy, the balance of immune responses, the clearance of cellular waste. Understanding this difference transforms how you approach your health.

The MILA Dynamic Intake

The R.E.S.T.O.R.E. MILA protocol begins with the Dynamic Intake - a comprehensive online assessment that captures your complete health picture. This is not a generic questionnaire. It adapts to your answers, asking follow-up questions based on the issues you identify.[34] The assessment contains six sections evaluating your health foundation, lymphatic function, immune function, mitochondrial function, thirteen body systems, and lifestyle factors - totaling 100 to 150 questions depending on your complexity.

Section A establishes your health foundation - demographics, health history, current diagnoses, medications, and contraindications that may affect your protocol. It identifies critical flags like blood thinner use, pregnancy, immunosuppression, or active cancer treatment that require special attention. Sections B, C, and D evaluate your three MILA pillars directly, generating scores for lymphatic, immune, and mitochondrial dysfunction based on primary indicators, secondary indicators, and contributing factors.

Section E uses a two-tier approach to assess thirteen body systems: gut and digestive, liver and gallbladder, kidney and urinary, hormonal, cardiovascular, respiratory, neurological, and cognitive, musculoskeletal, immune supplemental, infectious, skin, oral and dental, and mental and emotional. Core screening questions identify areas of concern, then Deep Dive questions explore those areas in detail. Section F captures your lifestyle foundation - including consumption of the Toxic Nine inflammatory foods and other lifestyle factors that directly impact MILA function.

Unlike conventional intake forms that focus on diagnoses and medications, the Dynamic Intake explores the terrain factors that create and perpetuate illness. It asks about toxic exposure history - occupational chemicals, mold exposure, heavy metals, pesticides, personal care products, water quality, air pollution. Most patients don't connect their symptoms to the toxic burden they've accumulated over decades - but the body remembers every exposure.

The assessment explores infectious history - not just acute infections, but chronic, persistent, or recurrent infections that reveal a terrain unable to maintain balance. Epstein-Barr virus. Cytomegalovirus. Herpes simplex. Lyme disease and co-infections. Parasites. Fungal overgrowth.[190] These infections don't just "happen" - they reveal a terrain that can't maintain balance.

It examines immune patterns: frequent infections, slow wound healing, autoimmune diagnosis or family history, allergies, food sensitivities, inflammation markers.[241] These patterns illuminate whether the immune system is under-functioning, over-functioning, or confused. It evaluates digestive function, energy and cognitive status, hormonal health, and emotional history - including major life events, trauma, and chronic stress periods that the nervous system doesn't distinguish from physical threats.[191]

From your responses, the assessment generates three MILA scores showing the level of dysfunction in each system: Mitochondrial, Immune, and Lymphatic. These scores provide objective measurement of your starting point and track your progress through subsequent phases. The assessment also identifies flags that affect protocol recommendations - factors like blood thinner medications, pregnancy, immunosuppressant use, or active cancer treatment that require special attention or modification.

The Questions That Reveal MILA Dysfunction

The Dynamic Intake asks questions designed to illuminate MILA dysfunction - questions that standard medical intake forms consistently miss. Here are examples of how specific questions reveal specific dysfunctions:

Lymphatic Indicators

Questions about morning puffiness, persistent dark circles, sock marks that last too long, chronic sinus congestion, and symptoms worsening with detox attempts all point to lymphatic dysfunction. The question "Do you experience post-exertional malaise - feeling worse after activity?" is particularly revealing, indicating both lymphatic congestion and mitochondrial involvement. Slow wound healing and swollen lymph nodes when not sick are primary lymphatic indicators that conventional medicine rarely connects to systemic dysfunction.

Immune Indicators

The assessment evaluates immune function through questions about autoimmune diagnoses, food reactions, chemical sensitivities, infection frequency, and symptom patterns.[241] "Do your symptoms come and go in cycles or flares?" suggests immune dysregulation. "Did your symptoms worsen after a major infection?" - often pointing to conditions like Long COVID or post-viral syndrome. Histamine-type reactions like flushing, hives, or headaches indicate immune imbalance requiring specific protocol modifications.

Mitochondrial Indicators

"Do you experience persistent, crushing fatigue that is not relieved by rest?" is a hallmark of mitochondrial dysfunction. Exercise intolerance - being unable to exercise or feeling much worse after - directly reflects cellular energy failure.[6] Brain fog, temperature dysregulation, post-meal fatigue, poor stress tolerance, afternoon energy crashes, and muscle weakness without clear cause all indicate that mitochondria cannot meet energy demands.[192]

Pattern Recognition

The power of the Dynamic Intake lies in pattern recognition. Individual symptoms mean little in isolation. But when morning brain fog that improves through the day combines with dark circles, puffiness, and worsening with detox - that's a lymphatic pattern. When crushing fatigue combines with exercise intolerance, temperature problems, and afternoon crashes - that's a mitochondrial pattern. When food reactions combine with chemical sensitivity, frequent infections, and symptom flares - that's an immune pattern. The assessment captures these patterns systematically, generating MILA scores that quantify dysfunction in each pillar.

The Fundamental Four: Targeted Testing

Beyond the Dynamic Intake, the Fundamental Four laboratory tests provide deeper insight into cellular function. These aren't random tests - they are specifically chosen to illuminate MILA dysfunction in ways that standard medical testing cannot.[193]

Comprehensive Nutritional and Metabolic Assessment

This assessment evaluates vitamins, minerals, amino acids, fatty acids, organic acids, oxidative stress markers, and toxin indicators.

It's not just about identifying deficiencies - it's about understanding how nutrients affect mitochondrial function, antioxidant capacity, neurotransmitter production, and detoxification pathways.[194]

The organic acids panel within this assessment is particularly revealing. It shows mitochondrial function markers - citric acid cycle intermediates that reveal whether cells are generating energy efficiently or stuck in anaerobic metabolism.[20] Elevated pyruvate and lactate indicate mitochondrial dysfunction - cells can't complete aerobic respiration and are forced into less efficient glycolysis. This finding explains why patients feel exhausted despite adequate nutrition.

Neurotransmitter metabolites like homovanillate and vanilmandelate reflect dopamine and norepinephrine metabolism.[195] Serotonin metabolite 5-HIAA reveals mood regulation capacity. These markers don't just indicate neurotransmitter levels - they show whether your body can produce and metabolize them properly. Detoxification indicators like glucarate and sulfate show whether phase II liver detoxification is functioning. Oxidative stress markers reveal the cellular "rust" accumulating when antioxidant systems can't keep up.

Comprehensive Methylation Panel

Methylation is the process of adding methyl groups to molecules - a simple reaction that underlies thousands of critical functions. It's how your body produces neurotransmitters, processes hormones, repairs DNA, creates antioxidants, and detoxifies chemicals.[197] When methylation fails, everything downstream suffers.

The methylation panel reveals genetic variants (SNPs) in genes like MTHFR, COMT, MTR, MTRR, and CBS that affect methylation efficiency.[196] These aren't "defects" - they're variations that require different nutritional support. It also shows functional markers like homocysteine and SAM/SAH ratio - indicators of whether methylation is actually happening regardless of genetics. You can have perfect genes but poor function due to nutrient deficiencies or toxic burden.

This panel explains why some patients react poorly to supplements that should help them. Many people take methylated B vitamins without addressing cofactor deficiencies, creating imbalances rather than improvements.[197] The methylation panel reveals whether the pathway is running efficiently or creating a metabolic traffic jam that backs up detoxification.

Comprehensive Gastrointestinal Assessment

The gut is simultaneously the body's largest immune organ and a major lymphatic hub.[198] When gut health fails, so does systemic immunity, neurotransmitter production, nutrient absorption, and detoxification capacity. This assessment reveals the complete picture of gastrointestinal function.

It evaluates microbiome diversity and balance - beneficial bacteria levels, pathogenic bacteria presence, fungal overgrowth, and parasites.[199] Diversity is key - a healthy microbiome contains hundreds of species working in concert. Loss of diversity allows opportunistic organisms to dominate. Inflammatory markers like calprotectin and lactoferrin indicate intestinal inflammation - a constant drain on MILA resources.[200]

The assessment includes digestive function markers showing enzyme production and fat absorption. It measures intestinal permeability through zonulin - a protein that regulates tight junctions between intestinal cells.[201] When zonulin is elevated, the intestinal barrier is compromised, allowing undigested food particles, bacterial endotoxins, and inflammatory molecules into the bloodstream. It also measures short-chain fatty acids - critical metabolites produced by beneficial bacteria that feed colonocytes and reduce inflammation.[202]

Comprehensive Food Sensitivity Panel

Food sensitivities are different from food allergies. Allergies are immediate IgE reactions - anaphylaxis, hives, swelling. Sensitivities are delayed IgG reactions that can take 72 hours to manifest, making them nearly impossible to identify without testing.[203]

Why does this matter for MILA dysfunction? Because every time you eat food your immune system reacts to, you trigger systemic inflammation.[204] The immune system creates antibody-antigen complexes that circulate in the bloodstream. The lymphatic system tries to clear them but becomes overwhelmed. Chronic exposure creates chronic immune activation - a constant drain on MILA resources that prevents healing regardless of other interventions.

Common culprits include gluten and wheat (not just for celiacs), dairy proteins, eggs, corn, soy, and peanuts.[205] Some patients discover they're reactive to dozens of foods - eating triggers immune responses at every meal. Their bodies are in constant battle mode, unable to focus on healing because they're perpetually fighting perceived threats from their diet.

Reading Your Body's Signals

Not everyone can afford comprehensive functional testing. A full Fundamental Four panel costs two to four thousand dollars. That's a barrier for many people seeking help. But your body constantly communicates its state through visible signs. Learning to read these signals provides valuable insight even without laboratory confirmation:

Dark circles under eyes: Not just from poor sleep. Dark circles indicate lymphatic congestion, particularly in the nodes draining the face and sinuses.[206] The darker and more persistent, the more significant the drainage problem.

Puffiness or edema: Fluid retention signals lymphatic stagnation. If your rings feel tight by evening, if sock marks persist long after removal, if your face looks puffy in the morning - your lymph isn't flowing properly.

Skin issues: Acne, eczema, psoriasis, and rashes aren't just skin problems. They're signs your primary elimination organs are overwhelmed, forcing toxins out through the skin.[207]

Tongue coating: A white or yellow film on your tongue reveals gut dysbiosis and impaired detoxification. The tongue should be pink with minimal coating. Heavy coating suggests fungal overgrowth or bacterial imbalance that mirrors what's happening in your gut.

Bowel patterns: Less than one bowel movement daily indicates toxin recirculation.[208] Hard, pellet-like stools suggest dehydration and slow transit time. Loose stools can indicate inflammation, dysbiosis, or food reactions. The gut should move waste out efficiently.

Energy crashes after eating: Post-meal fatigue reveals mitochondrial dysfunction and potential blood sugar dysregulation.[10] Food should energize you, not exhaust you. If eating makes you tired, your cells can't process nutrients efficiently.

Brain fog that worsens throughout the day: Accumulating fog suggests impaired glymphatic drainage - your brain's waste removal system isn't keeping up with metabolic demand.[23]

Chemical sensitivity: Reacting to perfumes, cleaning products, or exhaust fumes indicates phase II detoxification problems. Your liver can't conjugate and eliminate environmental chemicals efficiently.[209]

Exercise intolerance: Feeling worse after exercise - increased fatigue, brain fog, or flu-like symptoms - points to mitochondrial dysfunction and impaired cellular energy production.[175]

Temperature dysregulation: Always cold? Can't tolerate heat? Poor temperature regulation reveals mitochondrial insufficiency and thyroid-adrenal dysfunction. The body can't generate or regulate heat properly.

Slow wound healing: Cuts and bruises that take weeks to heal indicate poor circulation, lymphatic stagnation, and compromised immune function. The repair systems aren't working efficiently.

From Data to Direction

The Reveal phase culminates in synthesis - taking all the information from the Dynamic Intake, testing when available, and observation, and creating a personalized map of dysfunction. This map answers three critical questions:

Where is energy blocked? Mitochondrial dysfunction shows up as fatigue, exercise intolerance, brain fog, temperature dysregulation, and poor stress tolerance. The location and severity guide mitochondrial support strategies in later phases.

Where is inflammation unresolved? Immune hyperactivation appears as food sensitivities, autoimmune markers, chronic infections, allergies, and elevated inflammatory cytokines. The pattern reveals whether you need immune suppression (rare) or immune rebalancing (common).

Where is waste trapped? Lymphatic congestion manifests as puffiness, dark circles, skin issues, chronic infections, slow healing, and reactions to detox attempts. The degree of congestion determines how gently you must approach drainage.

The answers to these questions determine your starting point. Someone with severe lymphatic congestion must begin very gently with drainage. Someone with profound mitochondrial dysfunction needs different support than someone with primary immune dysregulation. This is precision medicine - not treating diseases with standard protocols but understanding individual dysfunction patterns and addressing them systematically.

Common Assessment Pitfalls

Even with the best intentions, several mistakes can derail the Reveal phase:

Rushing through the assessment: Take your time. Accurate answers lead to accurate results. If you guess or rush, your protocol will not fit your actual needs. Think about how you feel most of the time over the past few months, not just today.

Under-testing out of cost concerns: Trying to treat blindly to save money often costs more in the long run. You waste months on ineffective protocols and potentially harmful interventions. Strategic testing provides clarity that makes every subsequent dollar spent more effective.

Ignoring patterns in favor of isolated markers: Looking at individual lab values without considering the complete picture misses the forest for the trees. MILA dysfunction creates patterns - recognize the pattern, and individual markers make sense.

Rushing to treatment before completing assessment: The pressure to "do something" often leads patients to start protocols before fully understanding the terrain. This almost always backfires with wasted resources and discouraging setbacks.

Failing to assess drainage before planning detoxification: This is the most common and most dangerous mistake. No amount of testing will reveal how well your drainage pathways are functioning unless you specifically assess lymphatic flow, bowel transit time, and clearance capacity.

Understanding Empowers Action

The greatest gift of the Reveal phase isn't data - it's understanding. When you finally comprehend why you feel unwell, fear diminishes. The problem is no longer "mystery illness" or "just getting older" or "all in your head." It's a system out of sequence, waiting to be restored.

This understanding creates agency. You're not a victim of random bad luck. You're not broken beyond repair. You're experiencing the predictable consequences of a terrain that can no longer maintain balance - and terrain can be restored. Every patient whose story we've shared in this book experienced this transformation. Margaret, David, Gloria, Raymond, Evelyn, Helen - each reached a point where their dysfunction patterns finally made sense. That understanding became the foundation for their recovery.

The Reveal phase transforms you from passive patient to active participant. Your observations become data. Your history contains crucial clues. Your response to previous treatments guides current strategy. After completing the Dynamic Intake, you receive a detailed report analyzing your MILA dysfunction patterns, identifying your primary areas of concern, and providing specific next steps tailored to your situation.

This self-directed approach isn't just philosophically empowering - it's clinically effective. Studies consistently show better outcomes when people are active participants in their health rather than passive recipients of care.[210] You're more likely to follow through with recommendations you understand and help develop through honest self-assessment. You're more likely to notice subtle changes that guide protocol adjustments. You're more likely to achieve lasting results when you understand the why behind every intervention.

With your MILA patterns revealed, you're ready to begin active intervention. The next chapter addresses the Eliminate phase - where the real work begins. You'll discover why elimination must start with drainage, not detoxification, learning the critical distinction between mobilizing toxins and actually removing them from the body. The lymphatic system's central role as your body's drainage network will become clear, revealing how gentle, strategic support creates the flow necessary for toxins to leave rather than recirculate.

Key Takeaways

- The Reveal phase must come first because intervention without assessment leads to wasted time and money at best, and harm at worst - supplements that should help can make symptoms worse when given out of sequence.

- The MILA Dynamic Intake is an adaptive assessment that generates three scores showing dysfunction levels in mitochondrial, immune, and lymphatic systems, creating a personalized map that guides all subsequent intervention.

- The questions that reveal MILA dysfunction focus on function rather than diagnosis - when symptoms begin, how they fluctuate, what makes them worse, and energy patterns throughout the day.

- The Fundamental Four tests - nutritional assessment, methylation panel, gastrointestinal assessment, and food sensitivity panel - provide biochemical precision revealing mitochondrial function, detoxification capacity, gut health, and immune triggers.

- Your body constantly communicates dysfunction through visible signs including dark circles, puffiness, skin issues, tongue coating, bowel patterns, post meal fatigue, brain fog, exercise intolerance, and chemical sensitivity.

- Understanding your specific pattern of MILA dysfunction transforms you from passive patient to active participant, creating the agency and clarity needed for successful restoration.

Wondering where you are in the R.E.S.T.O.R.E. process? Scan the code below to complete Dr. Thoma's Dynamic Intake and discover which phase of healing your body needs most right now.

Chapter 10

E - Eliminate: Opening the Pathways of Flow

Natalie had been managing her Type 2 diabetes for eleven years when she walked into my office, frustrated and frightened. At fifty-three, this accountant who had always prided herself on doing everything by the book had watched her health deteriorate despite following every recommendation her doctors gave her.

"I take my metformin religiously," she said, pulling out a ziplock bag containing seven prescription bottles. "I added a GLP-1 medication two years ago. My endocrinologist just started me on a third diabetes drug. My cardiologist has me on a statin and two blood pressure medications. And my numbers keep getting worse. My A1C was 5.9 when I was first diagnosed - now it's 8.2 despite all these medications. How is that possible?"

Natalie's story was painfully common. She had gained forty pounds since her diagnosis, mostly around her midsection. Her ankles swelled by afternoon. She woke up multiple times each night to urinate. Brain fog made tax season increasingly difficult. Her joints ached constantly, and she had developed fatty liver disease that her gastroenterologist was "monitoring." Most troubling, she had recently been told she was showing early signs of kidney dysfunction - the dreaded complication that haunts every diabetic.

"I did everything right," she continued, her voice cracking. "I switched to whole wheat bread. I use artificial sweeteners instead of sugar. I eat low-fat yogurt for breakfast. I choose lean meats and avoid red meat. I use vegetable oil instead of butter. I even started drinking diet soda instead of regular. Why am I getting sicker?"

I looked at her food diary, and the problem became immediately clear. Every single "healthy" choice Natalie had made was actually feeding her disease. The whole wheat bread was spiking her blood sugar. The artificial sweeteners were disrupting her gut microbiome and insulin signaling. The low-fat yogurt was loaded with added sugar. The vegetable oils were creating inflammation in every cell of her body. She was following the standard dietary advice perfectly - and it was killing her.

"Natalie," I said gently, "your body isn't failing you. It's being poisoned - by the very foods you've been told are healthy. And until we stop that poisoning and open your drainage pathways, no amount of medication will reverse what's happening."

Her eyes widened. "But my doctors never mentioned anything about drainage or toxins. They just keep adding more pills."

"That's the problem," I replied. "They're managing symptoms while the underlying dysfunction continues. Your swollen ankles, your frequent urination, your brain fog - these are signs that your lymphatic system is overwhelmed. Your body is trying to eliminate toxins, but the pathways are blocked. We need to work in a specific sequence: first stop the toxic assault, then open drainage, and only then support your body's natural detoxification. This is the Eliminate phase of the R.E.S.T.O.R.E. MILA protocol - and it's the foundation everything else builds upon."

The Intention of the Eliminate Phase

The Eliminate phase is the foundation of the entire R.E.S.T.O.R.E. MILA protocol. Its intention is twofold: stop the flow of toxins into your body and open your drainage pathways so toxins can exit.[186] Without this foundation, nothing else in the protocol works properly.

The wellness industry has created an entire economy around "detoxification" - a market worth billions annually that promises transformation in a bottle. Health food stores dedicate entire aisles to detox products: liver cleanses, colon cleanses, heavy metal chelators, parasite purges, and green powders guaranteed to "eliminate toxic buildup." The promise is seductive - simple solutions to complex problems, quick fixes for years of accumulation.

But here's the fundamental problem these products never address: you cannot detoxify effectively while continuing to pour new toxins into your body, and you cannot mobilize stored toxins if your drainage pathways are blocked. It makes no sense to bail water from a sinking boat without first plugging the hole. And it makes no sense to force toxins out of storage when they have nowhere to go.

Your body already knows how to detoxify - it has been doing it since before you were born. What it needs is not more products to force toxin release. What it needs is for you to stop adding to the burden while opening the pathways so the toxins it is already trying to eliminate can actually exit.

The Danger of Out-of-Sequence Detoxification

I learned the importance of proper sequencing dramatically early in my career while working in a clinical laboratory. One afternoon, blood samples came through from students in a health sciences course who had all started an aggressive detox program together. Every single sample showed catastrophic results: severely elevated liver enzymes indicating acute hepatic injury, kidney markers suggesting renal failure, and metabolic derangements consistent with systemic toxicity.[211]

I ran the controls - they were perfect. I re-ran the samples - same results. These were not lab errors. These students' bodies were in crisis.

These young, relatively healthy students had overwhelmed their elimination pathways by mobilizing toxins before their drainage systems could handle the load. The program was aggressive: high-dose chelators, powerful binders, liver "flushers" - all taken simultaneously with no preparation and no drainage support. They were sick - fatigue, nausea, body aches, brain fog - but believed these were "healing crises" and kept pushing through. They had no idea they were poisoning themselves.

My recommendation was immediate: stop the detox program. Most recovered quickly once they stopped, but some had lingering effects for months. This experience crystallized a truth I have seen repeated countless times: if you mobilize toxins faster than your lymphatic system can clear them, your liver can conjugate them, your kidneys can filter them, and your bowels can eliminate them, you create an internal toxic crisis. The three pillars must be addressed in order.

The Three Pillars of Elimination

This phase typically lasts eight to twelve weeks and operates through three pillars that must be addressed in sequence. This order is not arbitrary - it reflects biological requirements that cannot be circumvented no matter how eager you are to feel better.

Pillar One: Stop the Toxins

Before you can eliminate what is already in your body, you must stop adding more. This means eliminating the Toxic Nine foods - sugar, wheat, corn, soy, dairy, peanuts, seed oils, alcohol, and chemical additives - that systematically destroy MILA function. [34] It also means reducing environmental toxic exposures from personal care products, household cleaners, air quality, and water. Any continued exposure undermines your progress. You cannot detoxify faster than you are being poisoned.

Pillar Two: Get Lymph Flowing

Your lymphatic system is your body's primary drainage network, collecting waste from every cell and tissue. But unlike your circulatory system, it has no pump.[212] It relies entirely on your activity to move fluid. Deep breathing, walking, hydration, and manual techniques create the pumping action that moves lymph through vessels and clears the pathways for toxin exit. Without flow, toxins have nowhere to go.

Pillar Three: Remove Toxins

Only after you have stopped adding toxins and opened drainage pathways can you safely support toxin removal. Targeted supplements - drainage remedies, binders, glutathione, and immunoglobulins - capture and escort toxins out of your body through now-open pathways.[213] Attempting removal before the first two pillars are addressed creates the toxic recirculation that makes people sicker.

Pillar One: Eliminating the Toxic Nine

The Toxic Nine foods must be completely eliminated - not reduced, eliminated - for the duration of the protocol. This is not a recommendation; it is a requirement. Any continued exposure undermines your progress.[187] The Toxic Nine include:

Sugar in all forms, including honey, maple syrup, and "natural" sweeteners. Sugar feeds pathogenic bacteria, disrupts blood sugar regulation, directly impairs mitochondrial function, and triggers inflammatory cascades throughout the body.

Wheat and gluten-containing grains damage the gut barrier by triggering zonulin release, causing intestinal permeability even in people without celiac disease. Gluten also triggers immune reactions and neurological inflammation.[201]

Corn and corn-derived ingredients including corn syrup, cornstarch, and corn oil - almost universally genetically modified and contaminated with glyphosate. GM corn contains Cry proteins that damage mitochondrial function.[214]

Soy in all forms acts as a potent endocrine disruptor that interferes with thyroid function, sex hormone balance, and contains compounds that inhibit nutrient absorption and burden the liver.

Dairy from any animal contains proteins that trigger immune reactions in many adults, particularly casein A1 found in conventional dairy, contributing to inflammation, congestion, and digestive dysfunction.

Peanuts are highly susceptible to aflatoxin contamination, a potent mycotoxin that damages the liver and immune system. They also contain lectins that can irritate the gut lining.

Seed oils including canola, soybean, corn, sunflower, safflower, and grapeseed are highly processed, oxidized, and inflammatory, disrupting cellular membrane function and promoting oxidative stress.[215]

Alcohol in any amount is directly toxic to mitochondria and the gut lining, depletes B vitamins and glutathione, disrupts sleep architecture, and requires significant liver resources to process.

Chemical additives including artificial sweeteners, colors, and preservatives are synthetic compounds that disrupt the gut microbiome, trigger immune reactions, and must be processed by the liver as toxins.

These are not arbitrary restrictions. Each of the Toxic Nine systematically damages MILA function through specific mechanisms: disrupting gut barrier integrity, feeding pathogenic bacteria, triggering immune reactions, overwhelming detoxification pathways, and poisoning mitochondria. For a comprehensive exploration of why each of these foods must be eliminated and what to eat instead, see Eat to Restore: The Food-

Based Path to Reverse Persistent Health Problems, Volume 2 of the R.E.S.T.O.R.E. MILA Series.

Beyond food, reduce environmental exposures. Switch to natural personal care products - what goes on your skin enters your bloodstream within minutes.[216] Replace chemical household cleaners with simple alternatives like vinegar, baking soda, and castile soap. Filter your drinking water - municipal water contains chlorine, fluoride, and often pharmaceutical residues. Improve indoor air quality with plants, regular ventilation, or HEPA filtration. These changes stop the ongoing assault so healing can begin.

Pillar Two: Getting Lymph Flowing

Your lymphatic system collects two to four liters of fluid daily from tissues throughout your body - fluid containing proteins, cellular debris, immune cells, pathogens, and toxins that must be processed and eliminated.[217] When lymph stagnates, all of this accumulates in the interstitial space where your cells live, creating an increasingly toxic environment. The cells literally sit in their own waste.

Hydration

Without adequate water, lymph becomes viscous and sluggish - like trying to flow honey through a straw.[218] Drink half to two-thirds of your body weight in ounces of water daily. For example, a 150-pound person needs 75-100 ounces daily. Start your day with 16 ounces of room temperature water before anything else. Add a pinch of high-quality sea salt to enhance cellular absorption. Drink four to six ounces every 30-45 minutes rather than large amounts infrequently - the body can only absorb about four ounces at a time. Stop significant fluid intake two hours before bed.

Deep Breathing

The diaphragm is your body's most powerful lymphatic pump. [219] When you breathe deeply, the diaphragm's movement creates pressure changes in the thoracic cavity that pull lymph from the lower body toward the thoracic duct where it enters the bloodstream for elimination. Shallow breathing - the norm for most stressed, sedentary people - dramatically reduces this pumping action.

Practice the MILA deep breathing technique two to three times daily: Lie down on a flat surface and place one hand on your chest and one hand on your stomach. Take a regular breath and while exhaling, push down on your stomach to fully get the air out. Then take a slow deep breath in, filling up your stomach with air and focusing on pushing your hand up. Continue the slow deep breath and focus on filling up your groin with air. Continue breathing in until you fill up your chest and neck with air as well. Open your mouth and exhale - the air should come out naturally without forcing. Complete five deep breaths, two to three times daily.

Movement

Walking is the most underrated lymphatic intervention. The rhythmic contraction of leg muscles acts as a peripheral pump that moves lymph through vessels.[220] Start with ten minutes daily, gradually building to thirty minutes. Focus on deep breathing while walking to maximize thoracic pumping. Rebounding on a mini-trampoline is exceptionally effective - the vertical acceleration and deceleration create pumping action throughout the entire lymphatic system. Even gentle bouncing without feet leaving the surface is beneficial. Yoga twists and inversions also help, with legs-up-the-wall for ten minutes dramatically improving lymphatic return from lower extremities.

Manual Techniques

Physical manipulation of lymphatic vessels can dramatically improve drainage.[221] Dry brushing before showering stimulates superficial lymphatic vessels - use a natural bristle brush and stroke toward the heart, starting at the feet and working up. The entire process takes five to ten minutes. Castor oil packs provide profound lymphatic support - saturate flannel with organic castor oil, place over the liver area on the right side of abdomen below the ribs, cover with plastic wrap, apply heat for 30-60 minutes, three to four times weekly. Professional lymphatic drainage massage is the gold standard but should wait until you have established baseline flow through the foundational interventions.

Pillar Three: Supporting Toxin Removal

The third pillar - removing toxins - is supported by targeted supplements that work together as a system. These supplements enhance what lifestyle practices make possible but cannot replace them. You cannot supplement your way around blocked drainage or ongoing toxic exposure. Follow the dosing on product labels and your personalized MILA report directions.

Lymphatic drainage supplement: Stimulates your lymphatic system to move and drain more effectively, supporting the body's natural ability to clear waste from tissues and move it toward elimination. Many people notice reduced puffiness, clearer sinuses, and improved energy within the first few weeks. Continue throughout the Eliminate phase and longer if lymphatic symptoms persist.

Glutathione: Called the "master antioxidant" because it is essential for nearly every detoxification process in your body.[177] It protects your cells from oxidative damage during the elimination process, supports your liver in processing toxins, and helps regenerate other antioxidants like vitamins C and E. Most people with chronic health issues have depleted glutathione levels. Supplementation in liposomal or S-acetyl form ensures optimal absorption. Continue throughout the entire protocol.

Binder: Attaches to toxins in your digestive tract and carries them out through your stool.[178] Without a binder, toxins released during elimination can be reabsorbed in your gut through a process called enterohepatic recirculation - making you feel worse rather than better. A good binder captures a wide range of toxins including heavy metals, mycotoxins, and environmental chemicals. Take at least two hours away from food, other supplements, and medications. Ensure you have one to two daily bowel movements before adding binders.

Immunoglobulin support: Provides concentrated immunoglobulins that bind to toxins, bacteria, and inflammatory compounds in your digestive tract.[179] By calming immune reactions in the gut, it reduces food sensitivities and supports gut barrier function. May be discontinued when gut reactivity and food sensitivities resolve.

Practical Implementation

The Eliminate phase typically lasts eight to twelve weeks and follows a specific sequence designed to address the three pillars safely and progressively.

Weeks 1-2: Stop the Assault and Establish Flow. Completely eliminate the Toxic Nine foods - no exceptions, no cheating. Begin reducing environmental toxic exposures. Start hydration protocol. Begin drainage supplement, glutathione, and immunoglobulins. Start gentle movement of ten minutes walking daily and deep breathing exercises two to three times daily. Add dry brushing before showers.

Weeks 3-4: Enhance Drainage. Increase movement to 15-20 minutes daily. Add castor oil packs three times weekly. Ensure one to two daily bowel movements before adding binder - this is critical. Introduce binder at bedtime, away from other supplements. Consider professional lymphatic massage if needed and tolerated.

Weeks 5-8: Optimize and Maintain. Continue all practices and supplements as directed in your MILA report. Monitor energy, mental clarity, and digestion for improvement. Add gentle sauna therapy of 15-20 minutes, two to three times weekly, if drainage remains open and tolerated.

Weeks 9-12: Assess and Prepare. Complete MILA Progress Assessment to measure improvement. Evaluate readiness for transition to Strengthen phase. Continue all foundational practices - they remain essential throughout the protocol and beyond.

When to Advance

You are ready to advance when you have completed eight to twelve weeks in the Eliminate phase, your MILA Progress Assessment shows improvement in your scores, you are tolerating the supplements well without significant detox reactions, you have one to two daily bowel movements, and you have consistently implemented the lifestyle practices.

Positive signs of progress include increased energy, improved mental clarity, better sleep, reduced puffiness, clearer skin, normalized digestion, and enhanced exercise tolerance. Most people notice these improvements gradually over the eight-to-twelve-week period.

Stay longer if you experience worsening fatigue, increased brain fog, headaches, nausea, body aches, anxiety, insomnia, or skin breakouts when attempting to progress. These warning signs indicate your drainage pathways are not fully open. If these symptoms occur, slow down - reduce binders, focus more on the first two pillars, and give your body more time. The goal is never to force elimination. The goal is to create conditions where elimination happens naturally, safely, and sustainably.

Natalie's Transformation

The first two weeks were the hardest for Natalie. Eliminating the foods she had believed were healthy - the whole wheat, the low-fat dairy, the vegetable oils, the artificial sweeteners - required completely rethinking everything she knew about nutrition. But by week three, something remarkable happened.

"My ankles," she said at her one-month follow-up, lifting her pant legs to show me. "Look - I can see my ankle bones again. I haven't seen them in years." The swelling that had plagued her for a decade was resolving as her lymphatic system finally began draining properly.

By week eight, her fasting glucose had dropped from 186 to 124 - without adding any new medications. Her blood pressure had normalized enough that her cardiologist reduced one of her medications. The brain fog that had made tax season a nightmare was lifting. She was sleeping through the night for the first time in years, no longer waking to urinate multiple times.

At twelve weeks, Natalie's transformation was undeniable. Her A1C had dropped from 8.2 to 6.4. She had lost eighteen pounds without counting a single calorie. Her fatty liver enzymes had improved significantly. Her kidney function markers, which had been trending in the wrong direction for years, had stabilized and even slightly improved. Her endocrinologist was cautiously optimistic about eventually reducing her diabetes medications.

"I was doing everything my doctors told me," Natalie reflected, tears in her eyes. "Whole grains, low-fat, artificial sweeteners, vegetable oils. Every single one of those recommendations was making me sicker. The foods I thought were saving me were actually poisoning me. And nobody told me about drainage - about why my body couldn't eliminate the toxins even when I tried to eat better. The sequence matters. You have to stop the poison, open the drains, and then support elimination. In that order."

With drainage pathways now open and the body's elimination systems functioning, we turn to the Strengthen phase - where we address the immune dysregulation that perpetuates chronic illness. The immune system, once calmed from the burden of constant toxic assault and given proper drainage support, becomes ready for the targeted regulation that restores balance between defense and tolerance.

Key Takeaways

- The Eliminate phase operates through three pillars that must be addressed in sequence: first stop the toxins coming in through Toxic Nine food elimination and reduced environmental exposures, then get lymph flowing through hydration, breathing, movement, and manual techniques, and finally support toxin removal with targeted supplements.

- You cannot detoxify effectively while continuing to pour new toxins into your body - eliminating the Toxic Nine foods stops the ongoing assault so healing can begin, plugging the hole before you try to bail water from the sinking boat.

- The lymphatic system has no central pump and relies entirely on your activity to move fluid - hydration keeps lymph thin, deep breathing creates the most powerful pumping action, movement activates muscle contractions, and manual techniques stimulate vessel flow.

- Four supplements work together to support toxin removal once drainage is open: lymphatic drainage supplement to enhance flow, glutathione for cellular protection, binders to capture toxins in the gut, and immunoglobulins to calm gut immune reactions.

- The Eliminate phase typically lasts eight to twelve weeks; advance when MILA scores improve, you tolerate supplements well, have one to two daily bowel movements, and experience increased energy and mental clarity; remain longer if you experience worsening symptoms when attempting to progress.

- The body knows how to detoxify - it has been doing it since before you were born - but it can only do so effectively when you stop adding toxins, open drainage pathways, and then support removal in that specific order.

For a more thorough understanding of the nutrition that supports every phase of the R.E.S.T.O.R.E. protocol, I direct you to my book Eat to Restore, a comprehensive dietary guide for terrain restoration.

Chapter 11

S - Strengthen: Restoring Immune Intelligence

Marcus held up his hands, and I could see the damage rheumatoid arthritis had wrought over the past seven years. His knuckles were swollen and misshapen. His fingers curved at unnatural angles. At forty-nine, this former carpenter could no longer grip a hammer - or even open a jar without his wife's help.

"I've been on every drug they make," he said, his voice a mixture of exhaustion and frustration. "Methotrexate for five years. Then they added a biologic - the one that costs four thousand dollars a month. Last year they switched me to a different biologic because the first one stopped working. Now they're talking about adding a JAK inhibitor on top of everything else."

He pulled out his medication list: methotrexate, a TNF inhibitor, prednisone for flares, folic acid to counter the methotrexate side effects, omeprazole for the stomach damage from years of NSAIDs, and a statin because the inflammation had elevated his cardiac risk markers. Six medications to manage the disease and its treatment complications - and his joints were still deteriorating.

"My rheumatologist says my immune system is attacking my joints," Marcus continued. "So we keep suppressing it with stronger and stronger drugs. But here's what I don't understand - if we're suppressing my immune system so aggressively, why do I catch every cold that comes through? Why did I get shingles last year? Why do I have constant sinus infections? How can my immune system be overactive enough to destroy my joints but too weak to fight off a common cold?"

It was the right question the question that reveals the fundamental flaw in how conventional medicine approaches autoimmune disease. Marcus's immune system was not simply "overactive." It was dysregulated - attacking the wrong targets while failing to address genuine threats. The drugs were suppressing immune function across the board, but they were not teaching his immune system how to regulate itself. They were not addressing why it had become confused in the first place.

"Marcus," I said, "your immune system doesn't need more suppression. It needs education. Right now, it can't tell the difference between your joint tissues and foreign invaders. It's mounting a full-scale assault on your own body while simultaneously being too exhausted to fight actual infections. We need to teach it when to attack and when to stand down. That's what the Strengthen phase is designed to do."

The Intention of the Strengthen Phase

The Strengthen phase focuses on restoring immune intelligence. Its intention is not to boost or stimulate your immune system, but to teach it how to regulate itself - responding vigorously to genuine threats while tolerating harmless substances and turning off inflammation once the threat has passed.[225]

Modern medicine - both conventional and functional - makes the same fundamental mistake about immunity: they assume more is better. Boost immunity. Strengthen defenses. Support immune function. The language reveals the underlying assumption - that chronic illness results from weak immunity requiring enhancement. This is precisely backward.

In chronic illness, it is often not an issue of the immune system being weak - it is dysregulated. It is overactive in ways that cause harm, underactive in ways that allow opportunistic infections, and fundamentally unable to tell friend from foe. The problem is not insufficient immune response - it is unintelligent immune response.

Think about autoimmune disease. The immune system is incredibly active - producing antibodies, releasing inflammatory chemicals, mobilizing defensive cells. But this activity destroys rather than protects. The immune system attacks thyroid tissue in Hashimoto's, joint tissues in rheumatoid arthritis, the protective coating on nerves in multiple sclerosis, intestinal lining in Crohn's disease, insulin-producing cells in Type 1 diabetes. More immune activity makes things worse, not better.

Or consider allergies and food sensitivities. The immune system mounts vigorous responses to things that pose no genuine threat - pollen, pet dander, foods eaten safely by billions of people. Again, the problem is not immune weakness - it is immune overreaction. The solution is not immune stimulation. It is immune modulation - teaching the immune system to regulate itself.

This phase typically lasts eight weeks and builds on the foundation established in the Eliminate phase. With drainage pathways open and toxic burden reduced, your immune system now has the space and resources it needs to rebalance. Attempting immune modulation before drainage is established - while lymphatic channels remain blocked and toxins continue accumulating - creates temporary improvement at best.

The Core Principle: Modulation, Not Stimulation

The distinction between modulation and stimulation is critical and often misunderstood, even by practitioners.

Immune stimulation increases immune activity across the board - more antibodies, more inflammatory chemicals, more cell mobilization. This is appropriate for someone with genuine immune suppression: advanced HIV, post-chemotherapy, certain genetic immunodeficiency conditions. For these patients, the immune system truly is too weak and needs boosting.

Immune modulation teaches the immune system to respond appropriately - increasing activity against genuine threats while decreasing inappropriate reactions to harmless substances. [170] It is not about more or less immune function; it is about smarter immune function. The goal is an immune system that responds vigorously to genuine threats while tolerating the harmless substances it encounters daily.

Supplements marketed as "immune boosters" - echinacea, elderberry, astragalus, medicinal mushrooms, high-dose vitamin C - can actually worsen autoimmune conditions, food sensitivities, and chronic inflammatory states. They amplify an already-excessive immune response, adding fuel to a fire that needs to be contained rather than fed. What chronic illness patients need is immune education, not immune amplification.

This distinction explains Marcus's paradox. His immune system was simultaneously overactive against his own tissues and underactive against genuine threats. The immunosuppressive drugs were suppressing everything - the autoimmune attack and the protective functions. What he needed was selective regulation: calming the autoimmune response while preserving or even enhancing appropriate immune function.

Understanding Inflammation's Complete Lifecycle

Understanding immune intelligence requires understanding inflammation's complete lifecycle. Most people think of inflammation as a single event: something harmful shows up, the immune system attacks it, things calm down. But inflammation is actually a two-phase process, and chronic illness occurs when the second phase fails.

Phase One: Starting the Fire

When cells sense danger - infection, tissue damage, toxin exposure - they release inflammatory signals. These chemical messengers trigger the classic inflammatory response: increased blood flow causing redness and heat, fluid buildup causing swelling, and pain signaling. This phase is essential - without it, infections would overwhelm us, injuries would not heal, and damaged tissues could not be cleared and replaced. But inflammation was never meant to continue indefinitely. In healthy systems, phase one transitions smoothly to phase two within hours to days.

Phase Two: Putting Out the Fire

This is where chronic illness patients get stuck. Ending inflammation is not simply waiting for it to fade away - it is an active process requiring specific chemical signals and cellular behaviors. Scientists discovered molecules called Specialized Pro-Resolving Mediators, or SPMs - including resolvins, protectins, and maresins.[226] These molecules, made primarily from omega-3 fatty acids, actively signal the body to stop inflammation.

SPMs tell immune cells to stop producing inflammatory chemicals, stop recruiting more inflammatory cells to the area, switch from attack mode to repair mode, clear away debris, dead cells, and start rebuilding damaged tissue. Without enough of these resolution signals, inflammation never fully ends. The immune system stays activated. Tissues remain inflamed. Energy continues draining into immune activity rather than normal cellular function.

This is why omega-3 supplementation alone does not resolve chronic inflammation for most people - if the machinery for producing SPMs is impaired, which it is when mitochondria are dysfunctional and lymphatics are stagnant, simply providing more raw materials does not help. The factories themselves need repair first. This is another reason the sequence matters.

Strengthen Phase Lifestyle Practices

The Strengthen phase continues everything from the Eliminate phase - hydration, deep breathing, movement, dietary elimination of the Toxic Nine - while adding practices specifically designed for immune regulation. These lifestyle factors either support or undermine the regulatory mechanisms we are trying to rebuild. Supplements alone cannot restore immune intelligence.

The immune system does not exist in isolation. It is profoundly influenced by circadian rhythms, stress hormones, sleep quality, physical activity, and social connection. Each of these factors sends signals to immune cells, telling them whether to ramp up defensive activity or shift into regulatory mode. During immune restoration, we harness these signals intentionally to support the transition from hyperactivity to balance.

Light Exposure: The Master Immune Regulator

Morning sunlight is one of the most powerful signals for regulating immune function.[227] It sets your circadian rhythm, which controls the timing of immune cell activity throughout the day, and triggers vitamin D production in your skin. Get ten to twenty minutes of morning sunlight within thirty minutes of waking - go outside without sunglasses so your eyes receive the light signal. This is not optional - light exposure is a primary driver of immune timing and regulation.

Evening light reduction supports melatonin production and proper immune timing. Dim lights after sunset and minimize screen exposure before bed. The contrast between bright morning light and dim evening light establishes the circadian patterns that govern immune cell behavior.

Movement as Immune Medicine

Exercise is one of the most powerful immune modulators known - but the type and intensity matter enormously during immune restoration.[228] Gentle movement - walking, yoga, swimming, tai chi - supports lymphatic flow and promotes anti-inflammatory signaling. During this phase, avoid high-intensity exercise, which can trigger inflammatory flares in already-dysregulated immune systems. Think of "movement" rather than "exercise" - the goal is circulation and lymphatic flow, not performance or calorie burning. Continue building toward thirty minutes of gentle movement daily.

Sleep Optimization

The immune system does critical repair work during deep sleep phases.[229] Maintain consistent sleep and wake times even on weekends - the immune system thrives on predictable rhythms. Create a dark, cool sleep environment. Avoid screens for at least one hour before bed. Sleep optimization supports the immune rebalancing that occurs during rest - disrupted sleep perpetuates immune dysregulation regardless of what supplements you take.

Nasal Rinsing, Oral Health, and Environmental Factors

The nasal passages represent a primary entry point for pathogens and allergens. Daily nasal rinsing with saline solution - morning and evening - reduces the immune system's burden by physically removing irritants before they trigger responses. Mouth bacteria can enter your bloodstream and trigger systemic inflammation. Brush, floss, and clean your tongue daily. Poor oral health is consistently associated with elevated inflammatory markers and autoimmune activity.

Give your immune system fewer things to react to by reducing allergens in your home environment. Wash bedding weekly in hot water to eliminate dust mites. Use HEPA air filtration. Maintain humidity below fifty percent to discourage mold growth. These environmental modifications reduce the immune system's daily burden, freeing resources for proper regulation rather than constant reaction.

Loneliness and social isolation are profoundly inflammatory - studies show isolated individuals have significantly higher inflammatory markers than those with strong social connections.[230] Human touch, meaningful conversation, and community belonging all signal safety to the immune system, promoting regulatory function over defensive activation. This is not optional "nice to have" - it is biological necessity for immune restoration.

Strengthen Phase Supplements

The Strengthen phase supplements target inflammation and immune debris that have accumulated. These four interventions work synergistically to clear the battlefield, provide resolution signals, modulate immune pathways, and support regulatory cell function. Follow the dosing on product labels and your personalized MILA report directions.

Systemic Proteolytic Enzymes

Proteolytic enzymes - when taken between meals on an empty stomach - enter the bloodstream rather than being used for digestion.[231] Once in circulation, they break down inflammatory debris, immune complexes, excess fibrin, and other protein-based inflammatory material. Think of systemic enzymes as cleanup crews that clear the battlefield so the immune system can accurately assess the current threat level rather than continuously responding to accumulated historical damage.

For autoimmune patients like Marcus, this is particularly important. Immune complexes - clumps of antibodies bound to self-antigens - accumulate in joints, kidneys, and other tissues, perpetuating inflammation. Systemic enzymes help break down these complexes, reducing the inflammatory burden. Key enzymes include serrapeptase, nattokinase, bromelain, and papain. Take at least thirty minutes before meals or two hours after.

Omega-3 Fatty Acids

EPA and DHA from fish oil serve as precursors to those critical SPMs - the molecules that actively resolve inflammation.[9] Without adequate omega-3 fatty acids, the body literally cannot produce the chemical signals needed to turn off inflammation. It is like trying to stop a war when you cannot communicate the ceasefire order.

Most Americans consume omega-6 fatty acids from vegetable oils, grain-fed meat, and processed foods in vastly excessive amounts relative to omega-3s. Historical ratios were likely two-to-one or four-to-one omega-6 to omega-3. Modern Western diets often reach fifteen-to-one or even twenty-to-one. This imbalance biases the immune system toward inflammation and away from resolution. Therapeutic doses typically range from two to four grams of combined EPA and DHA daily. Quality matters enormously - rancid fish oil is pro-inflammatory, defeating the purpose.

Advanced Inflammatory Support

This is a full-spectrum botanical formula designed to help the body maintain a healthy inflammatory response. It contains a naturally balanced matrix of plant-derived polyphenols, protective oils, and bioactive proteins that work together to support antioxidant defenses, cellular resilience, and immune balance.[232] Unlike pharmaceutical anti-inflammatories which suppress symptoms without addressing underlying dysregulation, these botanical compounds work with the immune system's natural regulatory mechanisms.

Continued Glutathione Support

Glutathione, introduced in the Eliminate phase for detoxification, continues playing essential roles in immune regulation.[233] T-regulatory cells - the immune cells responsible for preventing autoimmune reactions and calming excessive immune responses - require adequate glutathione for proper function. When glutathione is depleted, regulatory T-cell function suffers, allowing unchecked inflammatory and autoimmune responses. Continue supplementation in liposomal or S-acetyl form throughout this phase.

Practical Implementation

The Strengthen phase typically lasts eight weeks, though individual variation exists based on the severity and duration of immune dysregulation.

Weeks 1-2: Initial Shifts. Continue all Eliminate phase practices and supplements. Add Strengthen phase supplements as directed. Add morning sunlight exposure of ten to twenty minutes within thirty minutes of waking. Begin nasal rinsing morning and evening. Subtle changes begin as systemic enzymes start breaking down accumulated inflammatory debris. Some experience temporary worsening as debris is mobilized and cleared. This typically resolves within days.

Weeks 3-4: Resolution Accelerates. More noticeable improvements emerge. Food reactions often begin diminishing in severity. Joint pain and muscle aches decrease measurably. Energy becomes more stable throughout the day. Sleep quality improves as nighttime inflammation decreases.

Weeks 5-6: Immune Memory Rewrites. The immune system begins "remembering" how to regulate itself rather than defaulting to overreaction. Foods that previously triggered reactions may become tolerable in small amounts. Environmental sensitivities often decrease. Inflammatory markers on lab testing often show significant improvement. Patients report feeling "more like themselves" - cognitive function sharpens, mood stabilizes, physical capacity increases.

Weeks 7-8: Consolidation and Transition. The immune system has established new patterns of response. Gains consolidate and stabilize. Energy is notably improved from baseline. The foundation is prepared for the next phase - Turbocharge. Complete MILA Progress Assessment to measure improvement and evaluate readiness for transition.

When to Advance

You are ready to advance when you have completed eight weeks in the Strengthen phase, your MILA Progress Assessment shows improvement in your scores, inflammatory symptoms have meaningfully decreased, food sensitivities have reduced, you are tolerating the supplements well, and you have consistently implemented the lifestyle practices. Energy should be notably improved from your Reveal phase baseline.

Stay longer if immune symptoms remain significantly active - persistent food reactions, ongoing joint pain, continued inflammatory flares, or if lab markers remain elevated. Some patients with severe or long-standing immune dysregulation need additional weeks. Attempting to advance before immune regulation is established leads to problems in the Turbocharge phase when we stimulate mitochondrial energy production - you cannot safely increase cellular metabolism in an inflamed system.

Marcus's Transformation

Marcus was skeptical when we began. He had been told his rheumatoid arthritis was a life sentence requiring ever-stronger immunosuppression. The idea that his immune system could be retrained rather than suppressed seemed too good to be true.

The first challenge was completing the Eliminate phase properly. Marcus had to acknowledge that despite his aggressive pharmaceutical treatment, his diet was still feeding inflammation. The "healthy" whole grain bread his wife made, the corn oil she cooked with, the low-fat dairy in his morning smoothie - all of it was perpetuating the inflammatory cycle his medications were trying to suppress. It was like running a furnace and an air conditioner at the same time.

But four weeks into the Strengthen phase, something unexpected happened. For the first time in two years, he went an entire week without needing his rescue prednisone for a flare. His morning stiffness, which had typically lasted three to four hours, was resolving within an hour. He could make a fist again - not tightly, but enough to grip a doorknob without pain.

At eight weeks, his rheumatologist was puzzled - and pleased. Marcus's inflammatory markers had dropped dramatically. His CRP, which had been chronically elevated at 18, was down to 4. His sed rate had normalized. His anti-CCP antibodies, a specific marker for rheumatoid arthritis activity, had decreased by forty percent. Most remarkably, he had gone six weeks without a single infection - after years of constant colds and sinus infections while on immunosuppressants.

"I finally understand what was happening," Marcus said in his twelve-week follow-up. "My immune system wasn't just overactive - it was confused. It was attacking my joints while simultaneously being too exhausted to fight actual germs. The drugs were suppressing everything, good and bad. What I needed wasn't more suppression. I needed to teach my immune system how to tell the difference between me and a threat."

By six months, working closely with his rheumatologist, Marcus had reduced his biologic medication by half. His joint damage had stabilized - no new erosions on imaging. He was back to light woodworking, making birdhouses for his grandchildren. The hands that had been too damaged to grip a hammer could now hold a chisel.

"I'm not cured," he acknowledged. "I still have rheumatoid arthritis. I still take some medication. But my disease is controlled in a way it never was before, and my overall health is better than it's been in years. I'm not just managing decline anymore - I'm actually getting better."

With drainage established in the Eliminate phase and immune regulation achieved in the Strengthen phase, the foundation is prepared for the next step in the protocol. Your lymphatic system is flowing. Your immune system has learned to regulate itself. Inflammation is finally resolving rather than perpetuating. Now we can address what many patients consider the core of their struggle: energy.

The mitochondria - those cellular powerhouses that have been locked in survival mode, diverting resources to immune defense rather than energy production - can finally come back online. In the next chapter, we explore the Turbocharge phase, where we directly support mitochondrial function. This is where the energy your body has been desperate for finally becomes possible. But it only works because we have done the preparation. Stimulating dysfunctional mitochondria in an inflamed system backfires - more energy means more inflammatory signaling, more reactive oxygen species, more tissue damage. With immune balance restored, we can safely add fuel to the fire without burning down the house.

Key Takeaways

- The immune system in chronic illness is not weak - it is dysregulated, overreacting to harmless substances while often failing to effectively address genuine threats; immune "boosting" typically worsens conditions by amplifying already-excessive responses.

- Inflammation is a two-phase process requiring active resolution signals, not just absence of triggers; without adequate omega-3-

derived Specialized Pro-Resolving Mediators, inflammation cannot properly resolve regardless of what triggers are removed.

- The Strengthen phase must follow the Eliminate phase because attempting immune modulation without first establishing drainage - while lymphatic channels remain blocked and toxins continue accumulating - creates temporary improvement at best.
- Four supplements work synergistically: systemic enzymes clear inflammatory debris, omega-3 fatty acids provide resolution signals, advanced inflammatory support modulates immune pathways, and glutathione supports regulatory T-cell function.
- Lifestyle factors including morning light exposure, gentle movement, sleep optimization, nasal rinsing, oral health, allergen reduction, and social connection are essential components of immune restoration - not optional additions.
- The Strengthen phase typically lasts eight weeks; advance when inflammatory symptoms have meaningfully decreased, food sensitivities have reduced, and energy has notably improved; remain longer if immune dysregulation persists to avoid problems in the energy-focused Turbocharge phase.

Chapter 12

T - Turbocharge: Restoring Mitochondrial Power

Vincent had built his reputation on stamina. At fifty-one, this emergency medicine physician routinely worked back-to-back twelve-hour shifts, managed a department of twenty-three staff members, and still found time to restore vintage motorcycles in his garage. His colleagues joked that he ran on coffee and sheer determination.

Then came the infection that changed everything.

"It wasn't even that severe," he told me, eighteen months after his initial illness. "Fever for three days, some fatigue, loss of taste for a week. I thought I'd bounce back. I returned to work after ten days. But I never recovered. Not really."

Vincent described post-exertional malaise so severe that walking to his mailbox left him bedridden for two days. Brain fog so thick he could no longer trust his clinical judgment - he had taken a leave of absence from the emergency department after nearly missing a critical diagnosis. Heart palpitations that appeared without warning. Sleep that never refreshed him no matter how many hours he spent in bed.

"I've seen every specialist," he continued. "Cardiology cleared me - my heart is structurally fine. Pulmonology says my lungs are normal. Neurology found nothing on imaging. Rheumatology tested me for everything autoimmune - all negative. Psychiatry suggested it might be depression or anxiety manifesting as physical symptoms. My colleagues, doctors I've worked with for twenty years, look at me like I'm making it up."

His voice cracked. "I'm a physician. I understand the body. And I'm telling you - something is fundamentally wrong with my cells. I can feel it. When I try to exert myself, it's like my body has forgotten how to make energy. I used to work double shifts without breaking a sweat. Now I can't walk up a flight of stairs. And nobody can explain why."

I understood exactly what Vincent was describing, because I had seen it hundreds of times - the post-viral syndrome that conventional medicine struggles to explain or treat. His mitochondria were not broken. They were locked in a protective state called the Cell Danger Response, and they would not come out of hiding until they received signals that it was safe.

"Vincent," I said, "your body is not failing you. Your mitochondria are protecting you. The problem is the danger signals that triggered this protective response have never fully resolved. Your cellular machinery is still waiting for the 'all clear' that never came. We cannot force your mitochondria to produce energy - that will only deepen their defensive posture. We have to create conditions where they feel safe enough to come back online."

The Intention of the Turbocharge Phase

The Turbocharge phase represents a critical inflection point in the R.E.S.T.O.R.E. MILA protocol. After eight to twelve weeks of opening drainage pathways in the Eliminate phase and eight weeks of immune retraining in the Strengthen phase, the terrain has fundamentally shifted. Lymphatic flow has been restored. Toxic burden has decreased. Inflammatory cytokines have normalized. The immune system has remembered how to regulate itself rather than remaining in chronic activation.[6]

The stage is finally set for what patients desperately wanted from the beginning but could not safely receive: direct mitochondrial support. This sequencing is not arbitrary - it reflects biological law. Mitochondria are exquisitely sensitive biosensors, constantly evaluating their environment for signals of safety or danger. When they detect threats - whether toxins accumulating in tissues, inflammatory cytokines flooding the extracellular space, or lymphatic stagnation preventing waste clearance - they initiate the Cell Danger Response, shifting from efficient energy production to defensive survival mode.

Attempting to force mitochondrial activation while danger signals persist does not boost energy - it triggers oxidative stress, inflammatory flares, and deeper fatigue. This is why Vincent had crashed every time he tried to push through his exhaustion, and why the mitochondrial supplements his naturopath prescribed made him feel worse rather than better.

His practitioners were not wrong that mitochondrial dysfunction was central to his illness. They were wrong about timing.

The Core Principle: Cell Danger Response

Before exploring how to restore mitochondrial function, we must understand why it fails in the first place. The conventional view treats mitochondrial dysfunction as simple mechanical failure - cofactor deficiencies, oxidative damage, genetic mutations. While these factors matter, they miss the fundamental dynamic: mitochondria do not just break down randomly. They shut down intelligently in response to environmental threats, initiating a coordinated protective program called the Cell Danger Response. [167]

Think of the Cell Danger Response as your cellular emergency broadcast system. When mitochondria detect danger - whether from infections, toxins, nutrient deficiency, psychological stress, or chronic inflammation - they do not simply produce less ATP. They actively reorganize cellular priorities, shifting from growth and energy production to survival and defense.

Metabolic Shift

Energy production switches from oxidative phosphorylation, the efficient process generating 36 ATP per glucose molecule, to glycolysis, which generates only 2 ATP per glucose.[234] This produces far less energy but allows cells to survive in hostile conditions. Your energy crashes not because your mitochondria are damaged but because they have deliberately downshifted into survival mode.

Danger Signaling

Mitochondria begin releasing ATP and mitochondrial DNA fragments into the extracellular space - not as fuel but as danger signals alerting the immune system. These molecular alarms trigger inflammatory responses, keeping the body in heightened defense. This explains why chronic fatigue often accompanies chronic inflammation - they are two sides of the same mitochondrial response.

Hormone Resistance

Cells reduce their responsiveness to hormones, particularly thyroid hormones and insulin.[235] This creates the pattern of "normal" hormone levels on lab tests while patients experience profound hormonal symptoms. The hormones are present, but cellular receptors are closed - another protective mechanism. I call this "cellular deafness" - the messages are being sent, but nobody is listening.

Cellular Isolation

Gap junctions between cells close, isolating each cell from its neighbors. In health, cells communicate constantly through these connections. In Cell Danger Response, the cells essentially "hunker down," cutting off communication to prevent danger spread. This cellular isolation contributes to the profound sense of disconnection and brain fog that characterizes chronic illness.

These changes represent intelligent adaptation, not pathology. They are designed to help cells survive acute threats. But when the threat never resolves - when toxins continue accumulating, inflammation persists, infections smolder - the Cell Danger Response becomes chronic. Mitochondria remain locked in defensive mode, unable to return to normal function even when provided with all the nutrients they need.

This is why simply providing mitochondrial nutrients without addressing the underlying threat signals fails. You are trying to coax a frightened animal out of hiding while the predator is still circling. The mitochondria need evidence of safety before they will resume normal function. The Eliminate and Strengthen phases provide that evidence - drainage flowing, inflammation resolved, immune system regulated - signaling to every cell that it is finally safe to come out of hiding.

Vincent's pattern was classic Cell Danger Response. His post-viral syndrome had triggered a protective shutdown that never resolved because the danger signals - chronic inflammation, immune dysregulation, lymphatic congestion - persisted long after the acute infection cleared. Every time he tried to push through, every time a practitioner gave him mitochondrial stimulants, his cells interpreted the increased energy demand as more danger and retreated further into defensive mode.

Turbocharge Phase Lifestyle Practices

The Turbocharge phase continues everything from previous phases - hydration, deep breathing, movement, dietary elimination, light exposure, sleep optimization - while introducing practices that stimulate mitochondrial biogenesis (the creation of new mitochondria) and mitophagy (clearing out damaged ones). [236] These hormetic stressors - mild stressors that make your body stronger by triggering adaptive responses - must be carefully calibrated during mitochondrial recovery.

Progressive Exercise

Movement challenges your muscles to create more mitochondria to meet increased energy demands. But during mitochondrial recovery, too much too soon triggers Cell Danger Response while too little fails to stimulate adaptation. Start with gentle walking and progress to moderate aerobic activity as tolerance improves. Exercise should leave you feeling energized, not depleted. If you need more than 24 hours to recover from activity, you have exceeded your mitochondrial capacity - scale back and build more gradually.

For patients with post-exertional malaise like Vincent experienced, this calibration is critical. The goal is to find the edge of your capacity without crossing it. Many patients find that walking, swimming, or cycling work better than high-impact activities during this phase. Track your response carefully and adjust accordingly. As mitochondrial function improves, your capacity will naturally expand - activities that once triggered crashes will become manageable, then easy.

Cold Exposure

Cold exposure activates brown fat and signals cells to produce more mitochondria for heat generation.[237] End your shower with thirty to sixty seconds of cold water, starting with cool water and gradually decreasing temperature over days and weeks as you adapt. Focus on breathing slowly and staying calm during the cold exposure - panicked breathing defeats the purpose by triggering stress responses. The key is consistency rather than intensity - daily brief cold exposure produces better results than occasional extreme cold.

Time-Restricted Eating

A 16:8 fasting pattern activates cellular cleanup processes including mitophagy - the selective destruction of damaged mitochondria.[238] Compress your eating into an eight-hour window, fasting for sixteen hours overnight. This intermittent fasting triggers autophagy, allowing your cells to clear out dysfunctional mitochondria and make room for healthy new ones. Some patients need to ease into this gradually, starting with a twelve-hour eating window and progressively narrowing over several weeks.

Heat Exposure and Senolytic Foods

Sauna triggers heat shock proteins that support cellular repair and proper protein folding.[239] Use sauna three to four times per week for fifteen to twenty minutes if available. Stay well hydrated and replace electrolytes lost through sweating. If sauna is not available, hot baths provide similar though less intense benefits.

Senescent cells - damaged cells that have stopped dividing but remain in tissues releasing inflammatory signals - contribute to chronic inflammation and impair tissue function. Certain foods help clear them: quercetin-rich foods like onions, apples, and berries; fisetin-rich foods especially strawberries; sulforaphane-rich foods like broccoli sprouts; and EGCG from green tea.[240] Emphasize these foods in your meals throughout this phase to support cellular cleanup.

Turbocharge Phase Supplements

Once the terrain is prepared - drainage flowing, immune system balanced, toxins reduced - we can begin the delicate process of coaxing mitochondria back to full function. This is not about forcing energy production through stimulation. It is about providing comprehensive support that addresses every aspect of mitochondrial biology. Follow your personalized MILA report for specific recommendations and dosing based on your assessment results.

Acetyl-L-Carnitine

This serves as the shuttle system that transports fatty acids into mitochondria for burning.[241] Without adequate carnitine, fats accumulate outside mitochondria while the engines inside starve for fuel. Beyond simple transport, it provides acetyl groups needed for the citric acid cycle and supports acetylcholine production for cognitive function. The acetyl form crosses the blood-brain barrier more efficiently than regular L-carnitine, supporting both physical energy and mental clarity.

Coenzyme Q10 (CoQ10)

CoQ10 is absolutely essential - it serves as the electron shuttle in the mitochondrial electron transport chain.[242] Without adequate CoQ10, the entire system backs up and electrons accumulate, generating damaging free radicals instead of ATP. The ubiquinol form is preferred over ubiquinone for those with chronic illness, as the conversion process may be impaired. CoQ10 also serves as a powerful antioxidant within mitochondrial membranes, protecting the very structures that produce energy.

B-Complex Vitamins

B vitamins serve as essential cofactors throughout energy metabolism.[243] B1 (thiamine) is required for pyruvate entry into the citric acid cycle - without it, glucose cannot be fully metabolized. B2 (riboflavin) forms FAD, a critical electron carrier. B3 (niacin) becomes NAD+, perhaps the most critical coenzyme in metabolism. B5 (pantothenic acid) forms coenzyme A, essential for the citric acid cycle. The key is using activated, bioavailable forms at therapeutic doses - methylfolate instead of folic acid, methylcobalamin instead of cyanocobalamin.

Magnesium

Magnesium is required for over 300 enzymatic reactions, but its role in mitochondrial function is particularly critical.[244] Every molecule of ATP must be bound to magnesium to be biologically active - it is actually Mg-ATP that cells use for energy. Without adequate magnesium, ATP cannot be utilized regardless of how much is produced. Bioavailable forms include magnesium glycinate for calming, magnesium malate for energizing, and magnesium threonate for cognitive support.

Continued Glutathione Support

Glutathione continues from previous phases, now serving critical mitochondrial protection.[245] Mitochondria maintain their own distinct glutathione pool, essential for neutralizing the reactive oxygen species inevitably generated during ATP production. Without adequate glutathione, increased mitochondrial activity generates oxidative stress that damages the very mitochondria we are trying to restore. This explains the paradoxical worsening that occurs on unsupported protocols - more energy production without antioxidant protection creates more damage.

Practical Implementation

The Turbocharge phase typically spans eight weeks. Here is what patients commonly experience:

Weeks 1-2: Subtle Awakening. Continue all Eliminate and Strengthen phase practices. Transition to Turbocharge phase supplements as directed in your updated MILA report - your supplement recommendations will change based on your Progress Assessment results. Begin cold exposure with thirty seconds of cool water at the end of your shower. Implement time-restricted eating in a 16:8 pattern. Initial improvements are often subtle - slightly better sleep quality, marginally improved morning energy, small increases in exercise tolerance. The mitochondria are beginning to respond but remain cautious, testing whether the environment is truly safe.

Weeks 3-4: Momentum Builds. Increase cold exposure gradually to 45-60 seconds at colder temperatures. Add sauna if available for 15-20 minutes, three times weekly. Progress exercise as tolerated. Energy improvements become more noticeable. Patients often report being able to do activities they could not tolerate before - walking farther, concentrating longer, recovering faster from exertion. Brain fog begins lifting as neurons receive more consistent energy supply.

Weeks 5-6: Breakthrough. For many patients, this is when the transformation becomes undeniable. Energy that felt forced or artificial in previous attempts now feels natural and sustainable. Sleep becomes more restorative. Physical capacity expands significantly. Mood stabilizes as neurotransmitter production normalizes with improved cellular energy.

Weeks 7-8: Consolidation and Transition. Gains consolidate and stabilize. The mitochondria have established new patterns of function. Energy levels plateau at a significantly higher baseline than before the protocol. Complete MILA Progress Assessment to measure improvement and evaluate readiness for the Optimize phase.

When to Advance

You are ready to advance when you have completed eight weeks in the Turbocharge phase, your MILA Progress Assessment shows improvement in your scores, energy has meaningfully and sustainably improved, you are tolerating the supplements and hormetic practices well, and you can exercise without prolonged recovery. Energy should feel natural rather than forced or jittery.

Stay longer if energy improvements are minimal, if you continue to crash after activity, if brain fog persists significantly, or if you cannot tolerate the hormetic stressors without setbacks. Some patients with severe or long-standing mitochondrial dysfunction need additional weeks. The mitochondria are still rebuilding trust with their environment - do not rush the process.

Vincent's Transformation

Vincent understood the science immediately - his medical training made the Cell Danger Response framework click into place. What he struggled with was patience. He had spent eighteen months trying to force his way back to health through willpower, and accepting that he needed to let his body heal on its own timeline, was the hardest part.

"I kept thinking like a doctor," he admitted. "Diagnose the problem, prescribe the treatment, expect results in a predictable timeframe. But my body wasn't responding to commands anymore. It needed to be listened to, not directed."

He completed the Eliminate phase in ten weeks, watching his swollen lymph nodes shrink for the first time since his illness. His wife noticed changes he could not see himself - less facial puffiness, better color, fewer dark circles under his eyes. The Strengthen phase brought his inflammatory markers down - his CRP, which had been chronically elevated at 12, dropped to 2. His food sensitivities, which had expanded to include dozens of foods, began contracting. By the time he began the Turbocharge phase, his terrain had genuinely shifted.

"Week three was when I noticed it," he told me at his follow-up. "I walked to the mailbox and back, and I didn't need to lie down afterward. It sounds ridiculous - a guy who used to work double shifts celebrating a walk to the mailbox. But that was the first sign that something was actually different. The same supplements that had crashed me before were now working. My body was finally ready to receive them."

By week six, Vincent was walking two miles daily without post-exertional malaise. His brain fog had lifted enough that he felt safe reviewing medical literature again. He was sleeping seven hours and waking refreshed - something that had not happened in nearly two years. His heart palpitations, which had been daily occurrences, became rare.

At three months post-Turbocharge, Vincent returned to the emergency department part-time. His colleagues noticed the difference immediately - the sharp diagnostic mind they remembered was back. His organic acids testing showed normalized lactate levels and balanced citric acid cycle markers. The mitochondrial dysfunction that had been so evident on testing eighteen months prior had resolved.

"I'm not running marathons yet," he acknowledged. "I may never run another marathon - and I've made peace with that. But I have my life back. I have my mind back. I can practice medicine again. And I understand now why nothing I tried before worked. I was trying to force my mitochondria to produce energy while they were still in survival mode. The sequence matters. You cannot skip the preparation."

Six months later, Vincent was back to full-time clinical work. He had even returned to his garage, finishing the vintage motorcycle restoration project that had sat untouched for two years. More importantly, he had become an advocate within his hospital, educating colleagues about post-viral syndromes and the R.E.S.T.O.R.E. MILA approach. "I was dismissed by specialists for eighteen months," he said. "I don't want my patients to go through what I went through."

With mitochondrial function restored, the stage is set for the Optimize phase. The brain, consuming twenty percent of the body's energy despite being only two percent of body weight, is exquisitely sensitive to mitochondrial function. When cellular energy production fails, the brain suffers first and most severely. Now that cellular energy production has been restored, we can address the complex neurological patterns that perpetuate illness - neuroinflammation, neurotransmitter imbalances, impaired glymphatic clearance, and the nervous system patterns that keep the body in defensive mode.

In the next chapter, we explore the Optimize phase - where we optimize brain function, mood, circadian rhythm, and the glymphatic system that clears waste from your brain during sleep. This is where many patients experience the final pieces clicking into place - the brain fog lifting completely, mood stabilizing, and cognitive function returning to levels they thought were lost forever. The energy foundation we have built in the Turbocharge phase makes this neurological optimization possible.

Key Takeaways

- Mitochondrial energy restoration must follow drainage optimization in the Eliminate phase and immune rebalancing in the Strengthen phase - not precede them; when mitochondrial supplements are given before the terrain is prepared, mitochondria interpret the stimulation as dangerous because environmental danger signals persist.

- The Cell Danger Response is not mitochondrial failure but intelligent protection - mitochondria deliberately downshift into survival mode when they detect threats, reducing energy production while increasing danger signaling, hormone resistance, and cellular isolation.

- Lifestyle practices provide hormetic stress that stimulates mitochondrial biogenesis: progressive exercise challenges muscles to create more mitochondria, cold exposure activates brown fat, time-restricted eating triggers mitophagy, heat exposure induces heat shock proteins, and senolytic foods clear damaged cells.

- Effective mitochondrial supplementation requires comprehensive support: fuel transport through acetyl-L-carnitine, electron flow through CoQ10, metabolic catalysis through B-complex vitamins, energy utilization through magnesium, and antioxidant defense through continued glutathione.

- The Turbocharge phase typically lasts eight weeks; advance when energy has meaningfully and sustainably improved, you can exercise without prolonged recovery, and energy feels natural rather than forced; remain longer if crashes continue or hormetic stressors cause setbacks.

- True vitality emerges not from forced stimulation but from creating conditions where mitochondria feel safe enough to produce energy efficiently, sustainably, and intelligently - working with your body's wisdom rather than against it.

Chapter 13

O - Optimize: Restoring Brain and Nervous System Function

Sandra had spent twenty-three years as a court reporter, her fingers flying across the stenotype machine at over 225 words per minute while simultaneously processing complex legal testimony. Her career depended on mental precision - capturing every word, every nuance, every objection in real-time with perfect accuracy.

Now, at fifty-seven, she could barely follow a simple conversation.

"They call it fibro fog," she said, her voice hollow with resignation. "Like it's some cute little side effect. But it's not cute. It destroyed my career. I made three critical errors in one deposition last year - three times I wrote the wrong word, words that changed the meaning of testimony. I've never made errors like that. I had to take disability leave. After twenty-three years of perfect transcripts, I can't trust my own brain anymore."

Sandra's fibromyalgia had been diagnosed eight years earlier, after two years of unexplained widespread pain, crushing fatigue, and sleep that never refreshed her. She had tried everything her rheumatologist recommended - Lyrica, Cymbalta, trigger point injections, physical therapy. The medications dulled the pain somewhat but added their own fog. The cognitive dysfunction had worsened steadily, year after year, until she could no longer do the work she loved.

"The pain I could manage," she continued. "I learned to work through it. But losing my mind? Watching myself become someone who can't remember what she read five minutes ago, who loses words mid-sentence, who walks into rooms and forgets why she's there? That's the part nobody warned me about. And nobody seems to know how to fix it."

Sandra had completed the Eliminate, Strengthen, and Turbocharge phases over the previous five months. Her pain had reduced dramatically - from a constant seven out of ten to an occasional three. Her energy had improved enough that she could get through a day without needing to lie down. Her inflammatory markers had normalized. But the cognitive symptoms persisted, stubbornly resistant to the interventions that had transformed the rest of her health.

"Sandra," I explained, "your brain is healing last because it requires the most. It consumes twenty percent of your body's energy while having no reserves to draw from. It depends on a specialized drainage system that only works during deep sleep - sleep that fibromyalgia has disrupted for years. Your body has built the foundation for brain healing. Now we need to give your brain the specific support it's been waiting for."

The Intention of the Optimize Phase

The Optimize phase represents the point in the R.E.S.T.O.R.E. MILA protocol where physiology becomes consciousness - where restored cellular energy finally powers restored mental clarity, where the biological healing of the body enables the neurological healing of the brain.[246]

After drainage restoration, immune rebalancing, and mitochondrial restoration, the body has built the metabolic foundation necessary to support the brain's intensive energy demands and unique detoxification requirements. This sequencing is critical: attempting to optimize brain function before establishing proper drainage, resolving inflammation, and restoring cellular energy production consistently fails because the brain's restoration depends on all these systems functioning correctly. You cannot optimize a brain that is energy-starved, inflamed, and drowning in metabolic waste.

The brain represents only two percent of body weight but consumes twenty percent of the body's energy and generates correspondingly massive amounts of metabolic waste.[247] Unlike other organs, the brain has no conventional lymphatic system - instead, it relies on the glymphatic system, a specialized fluid-exchange network that operates primarily during deep sleep to clear toxic metabolites, inflammatory debris, and protein aggregates.

This is why brain symptoms often persist even after other symptoms resolve. The body's lymphatic system clears waste continuously throughout the day. The brain's glymphatic system only functions effectively during specific sleep stages, under specific conditions of neurological calm. If those conditions are not met - if sleep is disrupted, if the nervous system remains hypervigilant, if inflammation persists in neural tissue - waste accumulates faster than it can be cleared. The result is brain fog, cognitive impairment, mood dysregulation, and the progressive neurological decline we have been taught to accept as inevitable. It is not inevitable. It is terrain dysfunction in neural tissue. And it can be reversed.

Why the Brain Heals Last

Understanding why neurological symptoms often persist longest requires understanding the brain's unique vulnerabilities and requirements.

No energy reserves: While muscles can store glycogen and fat tissue provides backup fuel for most organs, neurons cannot store significant energy.[28] They depend on moment-to-moment delivery of glucose and oxygen, with no buffer against supply interruption. When mitochondrial function fails systemically, the brain suffers immediately and severely - but it also takes longer to recover because there is no reservoir to draw from during restoration.

Blood-brain barrier complexity: This selective membrane shields neural tissue from toxins and pathogens in the bloodstream - but it also restricts nutrient delivery.[248] When the blood-brain barrier becomes damaged by chronic inflammation, toxins enter that should be excluded while nutrients that should enter become further restricted. Healing this barrier requires not just reduced systemic inflammation but active regeneration of the tight junction proteins that maintain their integrity.

Specialized detoxification: Most tissues rely on the lymphatic system for waste clearance, but the brain developed its own system - the glymphatic network - that operates on entirely different principles. Glymphatic clearance requires deep sleep, parasympathetic dominance, adequate hydration, and proper positioning. Modern life disrupts every one of these requirements.

Oxidative vulnerability: Neurons are extraordinarily vulnerable to oxidative stress.[249] Their high fat content, constant electrical activity, and intensive metabolic demands create continuous free radical generation. Without robust antioxidant defenses - particularly glutathione, which the brain requires in enormous quantities - oxidative damage accumulates faster than repair can address.

These factors explain why Sandra's body had healed while her brain lagged behind. The brain needed everything the previous phases provided - flowing drainage, balanced immunity, abundant energy - before it could begin its own restoration. Now those conditions existed.

Optimize Phase Lifestyle Practices

The Optimize phase continues all previous practices while adding specific interventions targeting the glymphatic system, circadian rhythm, and vagal tone. These lifestyle factors create neurological conditions where brain healing becomes possible. Without them, supplements alone cannot restore brain function.

Glymphatic System Optimization

The discovery of the glymphatic system revolutionized our understanding of brain health and disease.[23] For decades, scientists wondered how the brain - which generates enormous metabolic waste - managed to clear that waste without a lymphatic system. The answer was elegant: cerebrospinal fluid flows through channels around blood vessels, washing through brain tissue and carrying away debris.

But this system operates primarily during deep slow-wave sleep.[29] During wakefulness, brain cells are tightly packed, leaving little space for fluid flow. During deep sleep, brain cells shrink by approximately sixty percent, opening channels through which cerebrospinal fluid can surge. This nightly cleanse removes the metabolic waste accumulated during the day. Sleep deprivation does not just make you tired. It prevents your brain from taking out its trash.

Sleep position may also matter - research suggests side sleeping enhances glymphatic flow compared to back or stomach sleeping.[250] The lateral position appears to optimize the geometry of the glymphatic channels, facilitating more efficient waste clearance. If you currently sleep on your back or stomach, consider gradually transitioning to side sleeping.

For patients like Sandra with fibromyalgia, the glymphatic dysfunction creates a vicious cycle. Poor sleep quality prevents effective brain waste clearance. Accumulated waste contributes to neuroinflammation. Neuroinflammation worsens pain processing and sleep disruption. Breaking this cycle requires addressing sleep quality as a primary intervention, not an afterthought.

Circadian Rhythm Optimization

Your body's twenty-four-hour internal clock controls the timing of hormone release, body temperature, digestion, immune function, and cellular repair.[251] This master clock governs when you feel alert and when you feel sleepy, when your body repairs tissue and when it focuses on activity. Modern life constantly disrupts this rhythm through artificial light, irregular schedules, and late-night eating.

Get bright light exposure within thirty minutes of waking to set your circadian clock and trigger cortisol release for daytime alertness. This morning light exposure is the most powerful circadian signal - it tells your body that day has begun and sets the timer for sleep in fourteen to sixteen hours. Maintain consistent mealtimes within your eating window. Stop eating at least two hours before bed to allow digestion to complete before sleep.

Reduce artificial light exposure after sunset - dim lights in your home, avoid screens, or use blue-blocking glasses if screen use is necessary.[252] Blue light from screens signals daylight to your brain, suppressing melatonin and disrupting sleep onset. Keep your bedroom completely dark and cool at 65-68 degrees Fahrenheit. Go to bed and wake at the same time every day, including weekends, to reinforce your rhythm.

Vagal Tone Restoration

The vagus nerve connects the brain to virtually every organ system, carrying information in both directions. It is the primary pathway of parasympathetic activation - the "rest and digest" state that opposes the sympathetic "fight or flight" response.[253] When vagal tone is strong, the body can downregulate stress responses and enter the healing state where restoration occurs. When vagal tone is weak, the nervous system remains trapped in chronic low-grade activation, unable to fully relax even during sleep.

Deep breathing directly activates the vagus nerve and shifts the nervous system into parasympathetic mode.[254] Practice the MILA deep breathing technique twice daily - upon waking and before bed. Cold exposure also stimulates vagal pathways - even thirty seconds of cold water at the end of a shower helps. Humming, chanting, and gargling create vibrations that stimulate the vagus nerve where it passes through the throat. Social connection and positive emotional experiences strengthen vagal function over time.

Most patients with chronic illness have damaged vagal function - not from any specific injury, but from years of chronic stress, inflammation, and sympathetic dominance. Their nervous systems have forgotten how to rest. Even when danger has passed, they remain in vigilant mode, preventing the deep relaxation necessary for glymphatic clearance and neural repair. Restoring vagal tone is not optional - it is essential for brain healing.

Sleep Architecture Protection

Sleep quality matters more than sleep duration. You can sleep eight hours and wake exhausted if you are not achieving the deep sleep stages where restoration occurs. Alcohol, while it may help you fall asleep, suppresses deep sleep and REM sleep.[255] One drink can disrupt sleep architecture for an entire night. Even chronic stress, through cortisol's effects on sleep stages, can prevent the deep sleep that allows brain cleansing.

Prioritize sleep hygiene: consistent bedtime and wake time daily, a dark cool environment, no screens for one to two hours before bed, no alcohol within three hours of sleep, and no caffeine afternoon. Consider sleep tracking to monitor your deep sleep percentage and adjust practices accordingly.

Optimize Phase Supplements

The Optimize phase supplements support sleep quality, brain function, and neurotransmitter balance. With the foundational phases complete, the brain can finally utilize these supports effectively. Follow your personalized MILA report for specific recommendations and dosing based on your assessment results.

Sleep support formula: Promotes relaxation and healthy neurotransmitter balance for falling asleep and achieving restorative sleep stages. Unlike pharmaceutical sleep aids that provide sedation without true restoration, this formula supports natural sleep architecture. Take as directed in the evening, typically thirty to sixty minutes before bed.

Magnesium threonate: This specialized form of magnesium crosses the blood-brain barrier effectively to support brain magnesium levels.[256] Once in the brain, magnesium enhances GABA receptor sensitivity, amplifying GABA's calming effects. GABA is the brain's primary inhibitory neurotransmitter - it slows neural activity, reduces anxiety, and creates the calm that allows sleep. Studies show magnesium threonate improves cognitive function, memory, and sleep quality.

Neurological support remedy: Enhances glymphatic drainage and brain circulation, supporting the brain's waste clearance systems. It helps optimize the fluid dynamics that allow cerebrospinal fluid to wash through neural tissue during sleep, carrying away the metabolic debris that contributes to brain fog and cognitive impairment.

Continued glutathione support: The brain requires enormous quantities of glutathione to manage the oxidative stress generated by its intensive metabolic activity.[257] As neuroplasticity increases during the Optimize phase - as the brain actively rewires and repairs - antioxidant protection becomes even more critical. Continue liposomal or S-acetyl glutathione as in previous phases.

Practical Implementation

The Optimize phase typically spans six to eight weeks. Here is what patients commonly experience:

Weeks 1-2: Sleep Foundation. Continue all previous phase practices. Transition to Optimize phase supplements as directed in your updated MILA report - your supplement recommendations will change based on your Progress Assessment results. Implement strict sleep hygiene - consistent timing, dark room, no screens one to two hours before bed, no alcohol. Begin the MILA deep breathing practice twice daily. Initial improvements often appear in sleep quality - falling asleep faster, fewer awakenings, feeling slightly more refreshed upon waking.

Weeks 3-4: Cognitive Clearing. Brain fog typically begins lifting during this period. Word-finding improves. Mental processing speeds up. Patients often describe it as "the lights coming back on" - subtle at first, then increasingly noticeable. Mood often stabilizes as neurotransmitter production normalizes. Anxiety, particularly evening anxiety, tends to decrease.

Weeks 5-6: Mental Clarity Returns. For many patients, this is when cognitive function feels genuinely restored. Complex thinking becomes easier. Memory improves - both forming new memories and accessing old ones. Creativity returns. The experience of being fully present that had been missing becomes available again. Sleep becomes deeply restorative.

Weeks 7-8: Consolidation and Integration. Gains consolidate and stabilize. The brain has established new patterns of function. Cognitive capacity plateaus at a significantly higher baseline. Emotional regulation feels natural rather than effortful. Complete MILA Progress Assessment to measure improvement and evaluate readiness for the final phases.

When to Advance

You are ready to advance when you have completed six to eight weeks in the Optimize phase, your MILA Progress Assessment shows improvement in your scores, brain fog has meaningfully lifted, sleep is restorative, mood is stable, and you can think clearly and access words without difficulty. Cognitive function should feel natural rather than requiring constant effort.

Stay longer if brain fog persists significantly, if sleep remains unrestorative despite good sleep hygiene, if mood instability continues, or if cognitive function has not meaningfully improved. Some patients with long-standing neurological symptoms, significant blood-brain barrier damage, or history of head injury need additional weeks. The brain is rebuilding complex neural networks - do not rush the process.

Sandra's Transformation

The first two weeks were about sleep. Sandra had not slept well in eight years - the combination of fibromyalgia pain and prescription medications had fragmented her nights into restless stretches of light sleep punctuated by frequent awakenings. She could not remember the last time she had dreamed.

"The sleep hygiene changes were harder than I expected," she admitted. "No screens after eight o'clock meant no evening television, which had been my way of distracting myself from the pain. But I replaced it with reading actual books - something I hadn't done in years because I couldn't concentrate long enough. And the strict bedtime meant I couldn't stay up late hoping I'd eventually feel tired enough to sleep."

"Week three was when I had my first real dream in years," she told me. "I woke up and I could remember it - vivid, detailed, like dreams used to be. My husband said I'd actually been still during the night instead of tossing and turning. I didn't realize how bad my sleep had been until it started getting better."

By week four, she noticed changes in her thinking. She could read a full newspaper article and remember what it said. She could follow her husband's stories without losing track halfway through. The mental quicksand she had described was becoming solid ground again. Small things that had become difficult - remembering where she put her keys, following a recipe without rereading each step multiple times - began to feel automatic again.

At six weeks, Sandra did something she had not attempted in over a year: she transcribed a recorded conversation. It was just a podcast - nothing as demanding as legal testimony - but her fingers found the keys without conscious thought, and the words flowed from her ears to her hands the way they used to. She made no errors.

"I sat there and cried," she admitted. "Not because I was sad but because I was me again. The woman who could capture language at 225 words per minute wasn't gone. She was just waiting for her brain to heal."

At her three-month follow-up, Sandra had returned to work part-time, handling depositions two days a week. Her error rate was back to zero. Her rheumatologist was cautiously optimistic - her fibromyalgia was better controlled than it had been in years, with less medication than before. Her sleep study showed dramatic improvement in deep sleep percentage.

"They told me fibro fog was just something I'd have to live with," she reflected. "They told me to make lists and use reminders and accept my 'new normal.' Nobody told me my brain was drowning in waste it couldn't clear because I wasn't sleeping deeply enough to clean it out. Nobody told me there was a system for brain drainage and that mine wasn't working. Once I understood what was actually wrong, fixing it made sense. The brain heals last - but it does heal."

The Optimize phase reveals what may be the most important truth of the R.E.S.T.O.R.E. journey: the separation between mental and physical health is an illusion. Brain fog is not a psychological problem - it is a metabolic problem manifesting in neural tissue. Anxiety is not a character flaw - it is often a reflection of neurotransmitter insufficiency or vagal dysfunction. Depression is not a choice - it is frequently the consequence of neuroinflammation or mitochondrial failure in neurons.

Now, with drainage flowing, immunity balanced, energy restored, and brain function optimized, patients arrive at the final phases of R.E.S.T.O.R.E.: Repair and Everlasting. With the terrain fully restored, the body can finally address any remaining personalized repair needs and transition to sustainable maintenance for life.

Key Takeaways

- The brain heals last because it requires the most - it consumes twenty percent of the body's energy while having no energy reserves, depends on specialized glymphatic drainage that only functions during deep sleep, and is extraordinarily vulnerable to oxidative stress.

- The glymphatic system clears neural waste primarily during deep slow-wave sleep, requiring parasympathetic dominance, adequate hydration, and optimal sleep positioning - conditions that modern life systematically disrupts through artificial light, irregular schedules, and chronic stress.

- Sleep architecture matters more than sleep duration - deep slow-wave sleep enables glymphatic clearance while REM sleep processes emotional content; both are disrupted by alcohol, screens, irregular timing, and chronic stress.

- Circadian rhythm optimization through morning light exposure, evening light reduction, consistent timing, and meal scheduling creates the neurological conditions where sleep becomes genuinely restorative and brain function naturally optimizes.

- Vagal tone restoration through deep breathing practices, cold exposure, humming or chanting, and social connection shifts the nervous system from chronic vigilance to the parasympathetic state where healing occurs.

- The separation between mental and physical health is an illusion - brain symptoms reflect terrain dysfunction in neural tissue and respond to the same restoration principles that heal the body; cognitive decline is not inevitable aging but reversible terrain dysfunction.

Chapter 14

R-E - Repair and Everlasting: From Restoration to Resilience

Theresa sat across from me for her two-year follow-up, and I almost did not recognize the woman who had first walked into my office. Back then, at forty-eight, she had been swollen with inflammation, exhausted beyond measure, and terrified that the lupus destroying her kidneys would eventually claim her life.

Today, at fifty, she radiated health. Her face had lost the characteristic butterfly rash that had marked her for years. Her joints moved freely without the stiffness that had once made mornings a torment. Her eyes were clear and bright instead of the dull, fatigued gaze I remembered from our first meeting.

"My rheumatologist keeps using the word 'remission,'" she said, a smile spreading across her face. "She's cautious about it - she keeps saying lupus doesn't really go into remission, that I'm just well-controlled. But my ANA is in normal range now. My complement levels are normal. My kidney function has improved every quarter for two years. Whatever we want to call it, I haven't felt this good since before I got sick."

Theresa's journey had been one of the most dramatic I had witnessed. She had arrived taking hydroxychloroquine, methotrexate, prednisone, and a biologic medication. Her nephrologist had been discussing the possibility of dialysis if her kidney function continued declining. She had been told to expect a lifetime of immunosuppression and careful management of a disease that would never go away.

"The hardest part wasn't the protocol," she reflected. "It was believing it could work. I'd accepted that lupus was my identity now - that I was a 'lupus patient' forever. Learning to see myself as someone whose body could heal, whose immune system could relearn how to function normally? That took longer than any of the phases."

Now, two years later, Theresa maintained her health with a handful of supplements, consistent lifestyle practices, and the deep understanding of her body that the R.E.S.T.O.R.E. journey had given her. She had worked closely with her rheumatologist to reduce her medications as her labs improved. She was no longer on prednisone. Her biologic had been discontinued. She remained on low-dose hydroxychloroquine as a precaution, but even that was being discussed for potential discontinuation.

"I know lupus can flare," she said. "I'm not naive about that. But now I understand what triggers flares and how to prevent them. I know what my body needs. I'm not afraid of my immune system anymore - I've learned to work with it instead of against it."

The Intention of the Repair and Everlasting Phases

The final phases of the R.E.S.T.O.R.E. MILA protocol represent the culmination of everything that came before - and the transition from active treatment to sustainable health.[187] The Repair phase addresses any remaining structural issues now that the terrain can support tissue regeneration. The Everlasting phase transforms what you have learned into a lifestyle that maintains restored function for life.

By this point in your journey, you have accomplished something remarkable. You have opened drainage pathways that were blocked for years. You have cleared toxins that had accumulated for decades. You have rebalanced an immune system stuck in chronic dysfunction. You have restored mitochondrial function that had been locked in survival mode. You have optimized brain chemistry that had been struggling under systemic dysfunction.

The body rebuilds structure only after restoring function - this is biological law.[258] Attempting to repair tissues before establishing energy flow, immune balance, and neurological regulation invariably fails. The system simply lacks the resources and regulatory intelligence to maintain repairs. But once these foundations are secured, physical regeneration follows naturally.

This understanding contradicts much of conventional medicine. Traditional orthopedics often view structural problems as purely mechanical - torn ligaments need surgical repair, degenerated cartilage requires replacement, chronic tendinitis demands corticosteroid injections. These interventions focus on damaged tissue while ignoring the terrain that allowed damage to persist. Now, with terrain restored, your body can finally do what it has been trying to do all along: rebuild itself.

The Core Principle: From Protocol to Partnership

The journey through R.E.S.T.O.R.E. MILA has taught you something invaluable: your body is not your enemy. For years, you may have experienced it as unpredictable, unreliable, even hostile - betraying you with symptoms that seemed random and intractable. But now you understand the truth: your body was never broken. It was communicating.

Every symptom you experienced was intelligent signaling. Fatigue was not laziness - it was mitochondria locked in Cell Danger Response, conserving energy for survival. Brain fog was not aging - it was neuroinflammation from a congested glymphatic system. Pain was not random - it was inflammation from stagnant lymphatic flow and immune dysregulation.[167] Your body was doing exactly what it was designed to do in a terrain that could not support optimal function.

Now you possess something more valuable than any supplement protocol: understanding. You know that health is not the absence of symptoms but the presence of flow. You know that symptoms are not problems to suppress but messages to decode. You know that your body, given proper support, has extraordinary capacity to heal, adapt, and thrive.

Consider the typical trajectory patients follow: they arrive taking dozens of supplements prescribed by various practitioners over the years, spending hundreds of dollars monthly, yet still feeling unwell. Each practitioner had added their favorites without considering the whole. After completing R.E.S.T.O.R.E., these same patients maintain improved health with just a handful of carefully chosen supplements - a testament to the power of restored terrain over perpetual management.

I measure success not by how many supplements I can convince patients to take, but by how few they need while maintaining vibrant health. When a patient graduates to minimal supplementation, it means we have truly succeeded. The goal was never dependency - it was restoration of the body's innate capacity to regulate itself.

Repair and Everlasting Phase Lifestyle Practices

While supplementation becomes minimal in these final phases, certain lifestyle practices remain non-negotiable for maintaining restored terrain. These are not burdensome requirements - they are the natural behaviors your body was designed for, now integrated seamlessly into daily life.

Hydration

Half your body weight in ounces of clean water daily remains the foundation for lymphatic flow and cellular function. This is not optional - it is the medium through which every cellular process occurs. Continue starting your day with sixteen ounces of room-temperature water before anything else. Maintain the pattern of drinking four to six ounces every thirty to forty-five minutes rather than large amounts infrequently.

Movement

Daily movement that stimulates lymphatic drainage - whether walking, stretching, rebounding, or gentle yoga - prevents the stagnation that initiates dysfunction. Think "movement" rather than "exercise" - the goal is circulation and lymphatic flow. Thirty minutes of walking daily is sufficient for most people. Continue dry brushing before showers and consider maintaining castor oil packs one to two times weekly for ongoing lymphatic support.

Sleep

Seven to nine hours of quality sleep in alignment with natural circadian rhythms allows for glymphatic clearance and cellular repair that cannot occur during waking hours. Sleep is when your brain clears waste and your body rebuilds tissue. Maintain the sleep hygiene practices you established in the Optimize phase: consistent timing, dark cool environment, no screens before bed, and side sleeping to optimize glymphatic flow.

Stress Management

Some form of daily practice that shifts you from sympathetic dominance to parasympathetic recovery maintains the nervous system balance essential for MILA function. Continue the MILA deep breathing technique twice daily - upon waking and before bed. Cold exposure at the end of your shower, even briefly, continues to support vagal tone and stress resilience.

Real Food

Continue avoiding the Toxic Nine while eating primarily whole, unprocessed foods. This provides the nutrients and information your cells need to maintain optimal function without creating inflammatory burden. You have already proven you can do this - now it becomes your new normal. Some patients find they can occasionally tolerate small amounts of previously eliminated foods without triggering symptoms. Others discover they feel best maintaining strict elimination. Your body will tell you what works.

Seasonal Resets

Spring and fall represent natural times of transition when the body benefits from gentle drainage support - not the intensive protocols of earlier phases, but subtle assistance that maintains clear pathways.[259] A typical seasonal reset might include: two weeks of increased hydration; binders taken at bedtime for five to seven days; emphasis on drainage-supporting foods like beets, dandelion greens, and bitter herbs; and additional rest. Many patients also find it helpful to complete the progress assessment seasonally to monitor their terrain status and catch any emerging imbalances early.

Repair and Everlasting Phase Supplements

One of the most common questions I receive from patients completing the protocol is: "How many supplements do I need to take forever?" The question reveals a fundamental misunderstanding about what true healing means. If you need dozens of supplements indefinitely to maintain wellness, you have not actually restored terrain - you have just found a more sophisticated way to manage symptoms. Real healing reduces dependency, not increasing it.

By the time you reach these final phases, most patients find they can maintain vibrant wellness with a surprisingly minimal regimen. Follow your personalized MILA report for specific recommendations based on your assessment results.

Foundation multivitamin: A high-quality multivitamin provides foundational nutrients in bioavailable forms, covering common dietary gaps without mega-dosing individual nutrients. [260]

Omega-3 fatty acids: Continue omega-3 supplementation to maintain cellular membrane integrity and support the production of specialized pro-resolving mediators that keep inflammation balanced.[9] This is one supplement that provides ongoing benefit for virtually everyone.

Vitamin D3 with K2: These nutrients support immune regulation, bone health, and countless other functions. Target optimal ranges of 50-70 ng/mL for vitamin D, not just "normal" ranges.[261]

Structural support (Repair phase): For patients with specific structural repair needs identified through assessment, targeted peptides, enzymes, and minerals may be indicated temporarily to support connective tissue synthesis and tissue remodeling.[262]

That is for most people four to five supplements. Not forty. Not the shopping bag of bottles that many patients arrive with initially. Because when terrain is restored, the body maintains balance naturally.

Reading Your Body's Signals

With MILA literacy comes the ability to recognize subtle signals before they become significant problems. This early detection system allows for minor course corrections rather than major interventions.

Lymphatic congestion beginning: Slight puffiness in fingers or ankles, mild breast tenderness, subtle digestive changes.

Response: Increase hydration, add gentle movement, consider a few days of drainage support.

Immune imbalance starting: Increased reactivity to foods, slight seasonal allergies returning, minor skin changes. Response: Check for inflammatory foods that may have crept back in, ensure sleep quality is optimal.

Mitochondrial function declining: Energy dipping in the afternoon, exercise recovery taking longer, mental clarity wavering. Response: Assess stress levels, check sleep quality, ensure you are not overtraining.

Autonomic imbalance developing: Sleep becoming less restorative, stress resilience decreasing, mood becoming more variable. Response: Increase parasympathetic practices like deep breathing, reduce stimulant intake, prioritize recovery.

When you notice these early signals, you do not panic. You simply check your foundations: Have you been drinking enough water? Has stress been elevated without adequate recovery? Have inflammatory foods crept back into your diet? Has movement decreased? The answer usually reveals itself quickly, and the correction is typically simple.

When Symptoms Return

Even with excellent maintenance, life happens. Major stress, illness, travel, or simply aging can challenge your terrain.

Symptoms may occasionally return. This is not failure - it is feedback.

The difference now is your response. Instead of catastrophizing, you investigate with curiosity: What is my body trying to tell me? Usually, the message is clear. That international flight and time zone disruption stressed your system more than expected. The renovation project exposed you to more toxins than your drainage could handle. The family crisis required more resilience than your current resources provided.

Your toolkit for response is comprehensive. You know how to increase drainage support temporarily, add targeted supplements for specific challenges, modify diet to reduce inflammatory burden, increase practices that support nervous system regulation, and seek appropriate professional support if needed.

Most importantly, you know these occasional challenges do not erase your progress. The terrain you have restored has resilience. A temporary setback does not mean starting over - it means making adjustments and returning to balance.

Laboratory Monitoring

While body literacy becomes your primary guide, periodic laboratory assessment provides objective confirmation of terrain status. Annual or biannual testing might include a complete blood count, comprehensive metabolic panel, high-sensitivity C-reactive protein, and vitamin D levels.

These labs are not about finding problems to treat but confirming that terrain remains optimized. When results align with how you feel - as they typically will once terrain is restored - they provide reassurance and documentation of your progress. When results diverge from your subjective experience, they offer an opportunity for investigation before symptoms develop.

If basic testing reveals abnormalities or you notice terrain slipping in the wrong direction and have difficulty understanding why, additional testing from the Reveal phase may be warranted. Organic acids testing can assess mitochondrial function and neurotransmitter metabolism. Comprehensive stool analysis can evaluate gut health and microbiome status. Comprehensive hormone panels can identify endocrine imbalances. Food sensitivity testing can reveal immune reactions that may have developed. These deeper assessments are not necessary for routine maintenance but become valuable tools when course correction requires more information to guide the response.

The progress assessment at restoremila.com provides an additional layer of monitoring that captures terrain status in ways standard laboratory testing cannot. Completing the assessment seasonally - or whenever you notice symptoms emerging - gives you personalized guidance for course correction.

Theresa's Long View

Two years after completing R.E.S.T.O.R.E., Theresa remains in what her rheumatologist cautiously calls remission. She maintains her health with minimal supplementation, consistent lifestyle practices, and the deep understanding of her body that the journey gave her.

The path was not without challenges. Six months after completing the protocol, Theresa experienced what she initially feared was a flare - increased fatigue, mild joint stiffness, the beginning of facial flushing. In the past, she would have panicked, rushed to her rheumatologist, and likely been prescribed increased immunosuppression.

Instead, she paused and investigated. What had changed? She realized she had been under intense stress helping her elderly mother move into assisted living, sleeping poorly, skipping her morning walks, and eating convenience foods instead of her usual meals. She had stopped the deep breathing practice because she was "too busy." Her terrain was slipping, and her body was telling her.

Within two weeks of returning to her foundational practices - hydration, movement, sleep, real food, stress management - the symptoms resolved. Her labs, checked at her rheumatologist's insistence, showed no evidence of disease activity. What had felt like a lupus flare was actually her body's early warning system working exactly as it should.

"That experience taught me more than anything else," Theresa reflected. "My symptoms aren't random attacks from an enemy immune system. They're messages. My body was telling me I was pushing too hard, neglecting the basics, letting stress overwhelm my capacity. Once I listened and responded, the symptoms went away."

But more than physical health, she has reclaimed something she thought lost forever: confidence in her body. Trust that it will support her rather than betray her. Belief that her best years are not behind her but potentially ahead.

"I used to dread every lab result," she told me recently. "Every blood draw felt like waiting for a verdict. Would my kidneys be worse? Would my antibodies be higher? Now I actually look forward to my labs because they keep confirming what I already feel - that my body is working the way it's supposed to."

Her maintenance protocol is remarkably simple: the foundational supplements, consistent sleep, daily movement, real food, adequate water, and the wisdom to recognize when something needs attention. She completes the Dynamic Intake assessment seasonally to monitor her terrain status.

"The strangest part," Theresa reflected, "is how normal this all feels now. The practices that seemed overwhelming when I started are just life. I don't think about them anymore than I think about brushing my teeth. They're just what I do because I understand what my body needs."

Consider what Theresa's trajectory might have been without this intervention. Her lupus had been progressing toward kidney failure. The conventional path offered only escalating immunosuppression, eventual dialysis, and a shortened lifespan marked by disability. Instead, she chose to understand why her immune system was attacking her own tissues rather than simply suppressing it more aggressively. And the result is not just the absence of disease - it is the presence of vitality that surpasses what she thought possible.

Thinking in Decades

Everlasting Health is not about the next few months or even years. It is about the decades ahead. The terrain you maintain now determines not just how long you live but how well you live those years.[263]

Consider the typical American health trajectory: relatively healthy until fifty to sixty, then a gradual decline into chronic disease, increasing medications, decreasing function, and eventually years or decades of disability before death. This pattern has become so common that we have accepted it as normal aging. It is not normal. It is the predictable consequence of accumulated terrain dysfunction.

Now consider the terrain-based trajectory: maintained vitality through middle age and beyond, with minimal medical intervention, sustained function, and compressed morbidity - staying vital until very late in life, then declining rapidly rather than lingering in dysfunction.

This is how humans are designed to age when terrain is maintained. The Blue Zones research confirms this pattern in populations worldwide where terrain-supporting lifestyle practices are culturally embedded. In Okinawa, Sardinia, Costa Rica, and other longevity hotspots, people maintain function and vitality into their nineties and beyond - not through medical intervention but through the same principles you have learned: real food, daily movement, stress management, social connection, and purpose.

You now have the knowledge to create your own Blue Zone regardless of where you live. The practices may seem countercultural in a society organized around convenience, speed, and pharmaceutical management of symptoms. But you have experienced what happens when you align with your biology rather than fighting against it. You have felt the difference between managing illness and experiencing health.

This is not the end of your health story. It is the beginning of the best chapter yet - one written not by disease or dysfunction but by your informed choices, your body's wisdom, and the beautiful partnership between the two.

Welcome to Everlasting Health. Welcome to the life your biology always wanted to give you. Now live it fully.

Key Takeaways

- The body rebuilds structure only after restoring function - attempting tissue repair before establishing energy flow, immune balance, and neurological regulation fails because the system lacks resources to maintain repairs; the Repair phase succeeds precisely because the terrain has been prepared through all previous phases.

- True healing reduces dependency over time - most patients maintain vibrant wellness with a minimal regimen of foundational multivitamin, omega-3s, and vitamin D3 with K2, not the dozens of supplements that characterize symptom management approaches.

- Non-negotiable lifestyle practices form the foundation of Everlasting Health: adequate hydration for lymphatic flow, daily movement for circulation, quality sleep for glymphatic clearance, stress management for nervous system balance, and whole foods for cellular nourishment.

- MILA literacy transforms you into the primary authority on your own health - early warning signs become gifts rather than threats when you can recognize subtle signals and make small course corrections before dysfunction develops.

- Seasonal drainage resets in spring and fall honor the body's natural detoxification rhythms without requiring aggressive protocols - gentle support maintains the clear pathways you have established throughout the R.E.S.T.O.R.E. journey.

- The goal is partnership with your biology, not perfection - occasional indulgences will not undo months of healing when terrain is restored, but returning to chronic patterns will reactivate the pathways that led to illness; maintaining awareness while enjoying life creates sustainable health for decades.

Conclusion

Your Journey Forward

You have traveled a great distance to reach this point. From the opening pages where we met Margaret, exhausted and desperate after years of failed treatments, to the final chapter where Theresa maintains her lupus in remission through the simple practices she has made part of daily life - you have journeyed through a complete transformation of understanding about chronic illness and how to overcome it.

Along the way, you have met Natalie, whose Type 2 diabetes reversed when she stopped following the "healthy" dietary advice that was actually poisoning her. You met Marcus, whose rheumatoid arthritis improved when he learned to modulate rather than suppress his immune system. You met Vincent, whose post-viral syndrome resolved when he stopped trying to force his mitochondria to produce energy and instead created conditions where they felt safe to come back online. You met Sandra, whose fibro fog lifted when she finally achieved the deep sleep that allowed her brain to clear its accumulated waste.

Each of these patients arrived believing their body had failed them. Each left understanding that their body had been communicating all along - sending signals through symptoms that conventional medicine taught them to suppress rather than decode. Their conditions were not random misfortune. They were the predictable consequences of terrain dysfunction - and they resolved when that terrain was restored.

What You Now Understand

You understand that chronic illness is not a collection of separate diseases requiring separate specialists and separate medications. It is a unified dysfunction of the MILA system - the Mitochondria, Immune, Lymphatic Axis working together as an integrated whole. When this system functions well, health follows naturally. When it dysfunctions, chronic illness inevitably develops, regardless of the diagnostic label eventually applied.

You understand that the body is not a machine that breaks down randomly and requires external repair. It is a self-healing organism of extraordinary intelligence, constantly working to maintain balance and restore function. Symptoms are not malfunctions to be suppressed - they are communications to be understood. Pain, fatigue, brain fog, inflammation - each carries information about what the body needs.

You understand that sequence matters. The R.E.S.T.O.R.E. protocol works not because of any single intervention but because of the order in which terrain is addressed. Reveal the dysfunction through proper assessment. Eliminate toxic burden while opening drainage pathways. Strengthen immune regulation. Turbocharge mitochondrial function. Optimize brain and nervous system. Repair remaining structural issues. Maintain Everlasting health through sustainable practices. Skip a step or reverse the order, and the entire process fails.

You understand that the goal is not perfect adherence to a rigid protocol but partnership with your own biology. You have learned to read the early signals - the slight puffiness that indicates lymphatic congestion, the afternoon energy dip that suggests mitochondrial strain, the food reactivity that reveals immune imbalance. You know how to respond with small course corrections before dysfunction cascades into crisis.

The Paradigm Shift

The journey you have taken represents more than learning new information. It represents a fundamental shift in how you understand health, illness, and your relationship with your own body.

The old paradigm told you that chronic illness was your genetic destiny, that your body was defective, that the best you could hope for was management of inevitable decline. It told you to outsource your health to experts, to trust pharmaceutical interventions over your own experience, to accept that feeling unwell was simply part of aging. It divided your body into separate organ systems, each requiring its own specialist, each treated in isolation from the whole.

The new paradigm tells you something radically different. Your body wants to heal. It has been trying to heal all along. The symptoms you experienced were not attacks from a hostile immune system or failures of defective organs - they were your body's best attempts to communicate that something in the terrain needed to change. When you finally listened and responded appropriately, healing followed.

This paradigm recognizes that you are not a collection of parts but an integrated whole. Your mitochondria affect your immune system. Your immune system affects your lymphatics. Your lymphatics affect your autonomic nervous system. And your autonomic nervous system affects everything else. Treating one system while ignoring the others - the approach of conventional specialty medicine - can never achieve true healing because it violates the fundamental unity of your biology.

This shift changes everything. You no longer fear your body or dread its signals. You no longer feel helpless in the face of chronic illness. You have tools, understanding, and most importantly, a relationship with your own biology that transforms health from something that happens to you into something you actively participate in creating.

What Conventional Medicine Misses

Nothing in this book suggests that conventional medicine has no value. Emergency medicine saves lives every day. Surgical interventions repair damage that no supplement or lifestyle change could address. Pharmaceutical medications provide essential support for acute conditions and, in some cases, serve as necessary bridges while terrain restoration occurs.

But conventional medicine was designed for acute illness - infections, injuries, emergencies. It excels at crisis intervention. What it struggles with - and what it has largely failed at - is chronic illness. The same tools that save lives in the emergency room prove inadequate when applied to conditions that develop slowly over years and persist for decades.

The pharmaceutical approach to chronic illness typically involves identifying a symptom, finding a drug that suppresses that symptom, and declaring success when the symptom is controlled - regardless of what happens to the underlying dysfunction. Blood pressure medications lower numbers without addressing why blood pressure rose. Diabetes medications manage blood sugar without reversing the metabolic dysfunction that caused it. Anti-inflammatory drugs reduce pain without resolving the inflammation that generates it.

This approach creates patients who are never truly well but never obviously sick enough to demand different solutions. They accumulate medications over time, each addressing a symptom while potentially creating new problems that require additional medications. The average American over sixty-five takes four or more prescription drugs. Many take ten or more.

Few question whether this pharmaceutical dependence represents health or merely managed illness.

The R.E.S.T.O.R.E. approach offers a different path - not in opposition to conventional medicine but as a complement to it. Work with your doctors. Use pharmaceutical support when necessary. But simultaneously address the terrain dysfunction that allowed illness to develop in the first place. As terrain improves, medication needs often decrease. As MILA function normalizes, symptoms resolve naturally rather than requiring ongoing suppression.

The Road Ahead

Where you go from here depends on where you are in your journey. If you are reading this book while still struggling with chronic illness, the path forward is clear: begin the R.E.S.T.O.R.E. protocol. Take the Dynamic Intake assessment at restoremila.com to reveal your specific pattern of dysfunction. Follow the personalized recommendations through each phase. Trust the process even when progress feels slow.

Expect the journey to take time. Terrain dysfunction that developed over years or decades will not resolve in weeks. The phases are designed to be completed in sequence, each building on the foundation established by the previous one. Rushing the process - skipping phases or moving forward before your body is ready - typically leads to setbacks that require starting over. Patience is not just a virtue in this work; it is a requirement.

Expect challenges along the way. There may be temporary worsening as toxins mobilize or die-off reactions as pathogens clear. There may be moments of doubt when progress stalls or symptoms fluctuate. There may be pressure from well-meaning friends, family, or even healthcare providers who do not understand what you are doing. Stay the course. The patients whose stories fill this book all faced similar challenges. They succeeded because they trusted the process and persisted through difficulties.

If you have already completed the protocol and are maintaining restored health, your path is equally clear: continue the non-negotiable practices that support MILA function. Stay curious about your body's signals. Make small adjustments before dysfunction develops. Complete the progress assessment seasonally to monitor terrain status. Live fully, knowing that occasional challenges will not erase your progress as long as you return to the foundations that created it.

Whatever your current situation, remember that healing is not a destination but a direction. There is no finish line where you can declare victory and abandon the practices that created your health. But neither is there endless struggle - as the practices become habitual, they require less conscious effort. What once felt like discipline eventually feels like simply living in alignment with what your body needs.

The Ripple Effect

Your healing does not occur in isolation. As you transform your own health, you inevitably influence those around you. Family members notice your energy and begin asking questions. Friends wonder why you seem to be aging backward while they decline. Colleagues observe your resilience and want to know your secret.

You do not need to preach or persuade. Your transformation speaks for itself. Simply being willing to share what you have learned - when asked - can change lives. The mother who watches her daughter recover from chronic fatigue and asks what happened. The coworker who sees you refuse the office donuts and wonders why. The friend who notices you no longer complain about the aches and pains you used to share.

Every person who restores their own health creates ripples that extend far beyond themselves. Children learn by watching their parents. Communities shift one conversation at a time. The medical system, for all its resistance to change, eventually responds to patient demand for approaches that actually work.

You are part of a growing movement of people who refuse to accept chronic illness as inevitable, who understand that the body is designed to heal, and who have discovered through direct experience that a different kind of medicine is possible. Your success adds to the evidence. Your story joins the chorus of voices demanding better options than lifelong medication management of progressive decline.

A Final Word

Chronic illness stole years from many of the patients whose stories fill these pages. It stole careers, relationships, and experiences that can never be recovered. It created suffering that no one should have to endure, made worse by a medical system that too often dismissed their symptoms or offered only inadequate solutions.

But chronic illness also gave these patients something unexpected: a depth of understanding about their own bodies that most people never develop. A resilience forged through struggle. A gratitude for health that those who have never lost it cannot fully appreciate. And a mission to share what they learned so others might suffer less.

Margaret, who opened this book exhausted and hopeless, now helps other hospital administrators understand why their employees are struggling with chronic illness and what institutional changes might help. Natalie educates her fellow accountants about the metabolic impact of the office snack culture. Marcus has become an advocate for autoimmune patients in his community. Vincent trains medical students to take post-viral syndromes seriously. Sandra mentors other fibromyalgia patients through the R.E.S.T.O.R.E. process. Theresa speaks at lupus support groups about what terrain restoration made possible for her.

Their healing extended beyond their own bodies. It rippled outward into families, communities, and in some cases, into the very medical institutions that had initially failed them.

If you are currently struggling, know that your suffering is not meaningless. The knowledge you gain through your healing journey will serve you for the rest of your life and may serve countless others through your example and your willingness to share. The path is not easy, but it is clear. And at the end of it lies not just the absence of illness but the presence of vitality - the experience of what your body is capable of when every system functions as designed.

If you have already restored your health, know that maintaining it is both simpler and more important than you might imagine. The practices that healed you are the practices that will keep you well. They are not burdens to be endured but gifts to be embraced - the alignment with your biology that creates not just health but a quality of life that most people have forgotten is possible.

Your body has always known how to heal. It was waiting for you to provide the conditions in which healing could occur. Now you understand what those conditions are. Now you have the tools to create them. Now the journey forward is yours to walk.

Walk it well.

Continuing Your Journey

The R.E.S.T.O.R.E. MILA Series provides additional resources to support your healing journey:

Eat to Restore provides comprehensive guidance on the dietary changes that support terrain restoration, including detailed information about the Toxic Nine and what to eat instead.

Autoimmune Remission focuses specifically on autoimmune conditions and how the R.E.S.T.O.R.E. approach can support the immune system in regaining proper function.

Chronic Is Not Forever introduces the MILA framework and explains why chronic illness develops and how it can be reversed.

The Dynamic Intake at restoremila.com provides personalized assessment of your terrain status and generates specific recommendations for testing, supplementation, diet, activity, therapies, and lifestyle based on your individual patterns.

Whatever resources you choose to use, remember that the foundation of healing is not in any book or protocol but in your relationship with your own body. The tools exist to support that relationship, not to replace it. Listen to what your body tells you. Trust its wisdom. And never forget that the extraordinary capacity for healing that allowed every patient in this book to recover lives within you as well.

Your body is not your enemy. It never was. It is your partner in this journey, your most faithful ally, and the vehicle through which you will experience the vibrant health that is your birthright.

Welcome it. Trust it. And together, walk into the life your biology has always wanted to give you.

Ready to begin? Scan the code below to complete Dr. Thoma's Dynamic Intake and receive a personalized roadmap for your R.E.S.T.O.R.E. MILA journey.

Glossary

A

Adaptive Immunity: The branch of the immune system that develops targeted responses to specific pathogens through T cells and B cells, creating immunological memory for faster future responses.

Adenosine Triphosphate (ATP): The primary energy currency of cells, produced mainly by mitochondria. ATP powers virtually all cellular processes, from muscle contraction to nerve signaling.

Autoimmune Disease: A condition in which the immune system mistakenly attacks the body's own healthy tissues, causing chronic inflammation and tissue damage. Examples include rheumatoid arthritis, lupus, and Hashimoto's thyroiditis.

Autonomic Nervous System: The part of the nervous system that controls involuntary functions such as heart rate, digestion, and breathing. It consists of the sympathetic (fight-or-flight) and parasympathetic (rest-and-digest) branches.

B

Bioaccumulation: The gradual accumulation of toxins in body tissues over time, particularly in fat cells, leading to increasing toxic burden as exposure continues.

Blood-Brain Barrier: A selective barrier formed by specialized cells that separates circulating blood from brain tissue, protecting the brain from toxins while allowing essential nutrients to pass through.

Blue Zones: Geographic regions where populations have exceptionally high rates of longevity, characterized by lifestyle factors including plant-based diets, regular movement, strong social connections, and sense of purpose.

C

Calprotectin: A protein released by immune cells during inflammation, measured in stool to assess intestinal inflammation levels.

Cell Danger Response (CDR): A protective metabolic state triggered when mitochondria detect threats such as infection, toxins, or cellular stress. The CDR shifts cells from energy production to survival mode and becomes problematic when it persists chronically.

Central Sensitization: A condition in which the central nervous system amplifies pain signals, causing heightened sensitivity to stimuli that would not normally be painful. Common in fibromyalgia and chronic pain conditions.

Circadian Rhythm: The body's internal 24-hour clock that regulates sleep-wake cycles, hormone release, metabolism, and other physiological processes in response to light and darkness.

Cytokines: Small proteins released by immune cells that act as chemical messengers, coordinating inflammatory responses and communication between cells throughout the body.

D

Damage-Associated Molecular Patterns (DAMPs): Molecules released by damaged or dying cells that alert the immune system to cellular distress, triggering inflammatory responses.

Drainage Pathways: The body's systems for removing waste and toxins, including the lymphatic system, liver, kidneys, bowels, skin, and lungs. These pathways must be open before detoxification can be effective.

Dysbiosis: An imbalance in the gut microbiome characterized by reduced beneficial bacteria and/or overgrowth of harmful organisms, contributing to inflammation and impaired immune function.

E

Endothelial Dysfunction: Impaired function of the cells lining blood vessels, leading to reduced blood flow, increased inflammation, and elevated cardiovascular risk.

Epitope Spreading: A process in autoimmune disease where the immune system progressively attacks additional self-proteins beyond the original target, causing disease expansion over time.

F

Fibromyalgia: A chronic condition characterized by widespread musculoskeletal pain, fatigue, sleep disturbances, and cognitive difficulties, associated with central sensitization and mitochondrial dysfunction.

G

Glymphatic System: The brain's waste clearance system that removes metabolic debris and protein aggregates during sleep, using cerebrospinal fluid flow through channels surrounding blood vessels.

Glutathione: The body's master antioxidant, critical for detoxification, immune function, and protecting cells from oxidative damage. Levels decline with age and chronic illness.

Glycolysis: A less efficient metabolic pathway that produces energy (ATP) without requiring oxygen, yielding only 2 ATP per glucose molecule compared to 36 from oxidative phosphorylation.

H

Hemoglobin A1c (HbA1c): A blood test measuring average blood sugar levels over the previous 2-3 months, used to diagnose and monitor diabetes.

Hormone Resistance: A condition in which cells become less responsive to hormone signals despite normal hormone levels in the blood. Common examples include insulin resistance and thyroid hormone resistance.

I

Immunosuppression: Medical treatment that reduces immune system activity, used to prevent organ rejection and treat autoimmune diseases, but increasing susceptibility to infections and cancer.

Inflammaging: Chronic, low-grade inflammation that increases with age and contributes to age-related diseases and accelerated aging.

Innate Immunity: The body's first line of immune defense, providing immediate but non-specific responses to pathogens through barriers, immune cells, and inflammatory responses.

Insulin Resistance: A condition in which cells fail to respond normally to insulin, requiring higher insulin levels to maintain blood sugar control and eventually leading to Type 2 diabetes.

Intestinal Permeability: The degree to which the intestinal lining allows substances to pass into the bloodstream. Increased permeability (leaky gut) allows undigested food particles and toxins to enter circulation, triggering immune responses.

K

Key Takeaways: Summary points at the end of each chapter highlighting the most important concepts and practical applications.

L

Leaky Gut: A condition of increased intestinal permeability where the gut barrier becomes compromised, allowing bacteria, toxins, and undigested food particles to enter the bloodstream and trigger systemic inflammation.

Lymphatic System: A network of vessels, nodes, and organs that removes cellular waste, transports immune cells, and maintains fluid balance throughout the body. Unlike blood circulation, lymph flow depends on muscle movement and breathing.

M

Metabolic Syndrome: A cluster of conditions including high blood pressure, elevated blood sugar, excess abdominal fat, and abnormal cholesterol levels that together increase the risk of heart disease, stroke, and Type 2 diabetes.

Methylation: A fundamental biochemical process involving the transfer of methyl groups, essential for DNA repair, detoxification, neurotransmitter production, and energy metabolism.

Microbiome: The community of trillions of microorganisms living in and on the human body, particularly in the gut, which influence digestion, immunity, metabolism, and brain function.

MILA (Mitochondrial-Immune-Lymphatic Axis): The interconnected system of mitochondria, immune function, and lymphatic drainage that forms the foundation of health. Dysfunction in this axis underlies most chronic diseases.

Mitochondria: Organelles within cells that produce ATP (energy) through oxidative phosphorylation. They also serve as cellular danger sensors and regulate cell death, making them central to health and disease.

Molecular Mimicry: A phenomenon where foreign substances (such as bacterial proteins) structurally resemble human tissues, potentially triggering autoimmune attacks when the immune system confuses self with non-self.

Multimorbidity: The presence of two or more chronic conditions in the same individual, increasingly common with age and associated with complex medication regimens and poorer health outcomes.

Myalgic Encephalomyelitis/Chronic Fatigue Syndrome (ME/CFS): A complex, debilitating condition characterized by profound fatigue, post-exertional malaise, cognitive dysfunction, and sleep abnormalities, associated with mitochondrial dysfunction and the Cell Danger Response.

N

Neuroinflammation: Inflammation within the brain and nervous system, driven by activated immune cells (microglia) and contributing to cognitive decline, neurodegeneration, and mood disorders.

Neuroplasticity: The brain's ability to reorganize itself by forming new neural connections throughout life, enabling learning, memory, and recovery from injury.

O

Oxidative Phosphorylation: The primary metabolic pathway by which mitochondria produce ATP, using oxygen to generate 36 ATP molecules per glucose molecule - far more efficient than glycolysis.

Oxidative Stress: An imbalance between the production of reactive oxygen species (free radicals) and the body's ability to neutralize them with antioxidants, leading to cellular damage.

P

Parasympathetic Nervous System: The rest-and-digest branch of the autonomic nervous system that promotes relaxation, digestion, and tissue repair. Activated by the vagus nerve.

Post-Exertional Malaise (PEM): A hallmark symptom of ME/CFS characterized by worsening of symptoms following physical or mental exertion, often delayed by 24-72 hours and lasting days or longer.

Prediabetes: A condition of impaired blood sugar regulation where glucose levels are higher than normal but not yet high enough for a diabetes diagnosis. Affects approximately 96 million American adults.

R

R.E.S.T.O.R.E. Protocol: A seven-phase healing protocol addressing chronic disease through proper sequencing: Reveal dysfunction, Eliminate toxins and open drainage,

Strengthen immunity, Turbocharge mitochondria, Optimize brain function, Repair tissues, and maintain Everlasting health.

Regulatory T Cells (Tregs): Specialized immune cells that suppress excessive immune responses and maintain self-tolerance, preventing autoimmunity. Their dysfunction contributes to autoimmune disease development.

Remission: A state in which disease symptoms are significantly reduced or absent, which may be temporary or sustained depending on whether underlying dysfunction has been addressed.

S

Short-Chain Fatty Acids: Metabolites produced by beneficial gut bacteria during fiber fermentation, including butyrate, which nourishes intestinal cells and reduces inflammation.

Sympathetic Nervous System: The fight-or-flight branch of the autonomic nervous system that prepares the body for stress responses, increasing heart rate, blood pressure, and alertness while suppressing digestion.

Systemic Inflammation: Chronic, body-wide inflammation that affects multiple organ systems simultaneously, contributing to cardiovascular disease, diabetes, autoimmunity, and neurodegeneration.

T

Terrain: The internal environment of the body that determines susceptibility to disease. A healthy terrain resists illness while a compromised terrain allows disease to develop regardless of external factors.

Toxic Burden: The cumulative load of toxins stored in body tissues from environmental exposures, food, water, air, and personal care products over a lifetime.

Type 2 Diabetes: A metabolic disorder characterized by insulin resistance and elevated blood sugar, traditionally viewed as progressive but increasingly recognized as reversible through terrain restoration.

V

Vagus Nerve: The longest cranial nerve, connecting the brain to the gut and other organs. It regulates parasympathetic functions and plays a crucial role in the gut-brain axis and inflammation control.

Z

Zonulin: A protein that regulates intestinal permeability by controlling the tight junctions between intestinal cells. Elevated zonulin indicates compromised gut barrier function.

References

[1] Centers for Medicare & Medicaid Services. National health expenditure data: historical. CMS.gov. Published 2023. Accessed 2024.

[2] Centers for Disease Control and Prevention. Chronic diseases in America. CDC National Center for Chronic Disease Prevention and Health Promotion. Published 2023. Accessed 2024.

[3] Lerner A, Jeremias P, Matthias T. The world incidence and prevalence of autoimmune diseases is increasing. Int J Celiac Dis. 2015;3(4):151-155.

[4] Pulgaron ER, Delamater AM. Obesity and type 2 diabetes in children: epidemiology and treatment. Curr Diab Rep. 2014;14(8):508.

[5] Alzheimer's Association. 2023 Alzheimer's disease facts and figures. Alzheimers Dement. 2023;19(4):1598-1695.

[6] Naviaux RK. Metabolic features of the cell danger response. Mitochondrion. 2014;16:7-17.

[7] Emerging Risk Factors Collaboration. Diabetes mellitus, fasting blood glucose concentration, and risk of vascular disease: a collaborative meta-analysis of 102 prospective studies. Lancet. 2010;375(9733):2215-2222.

[8] Randolph GJ, Ivanov S, Zinselmeyer BH, Bhattacharya D. The lymphatic system: integral roles in immunity. Annu Rev Immunol. 2017;35:31-52.

[9] Calder PC. Omega-3 fatty acids and inflammatory processes: from molecules to man. Biochem Soc Trans. 2017;45(5):1105-1115.

[10] Picard M, McEwen BS. Mitochondria impact brain function and cognition. Proc Natl Acad Sci U S A. 2014;111(1):7-8.

[11] Buttorff C, Ruber T, Bauman M. Multiple Chronic Conditions in the United States. Santa Monica, CA: RAND Corporation; 2017.

[12] Anderson G. Chronic Care: Making the Case for Ongoing Care. Princeton, NJ: Robert Wood Johnson Foundation; 2010.

[13] Centers for Disease Control and Prevention. National Diabetes Statistics Report 2022. Atlanta, GA: US Department of Health and Human Services; 2022.

[14] Tsao CW, Aday AW, Almarzooq ZI, et al. Heart disease and stroke statistics - 2023 update: a report from the American Heart Association. Circulation. 2023;147(8):e93-e621.

[15] Tinetti ME, Fried TR, Boyd CM. Designing health care for the most common chronic condition - multimorbidity. JAMA. 2012;307(23):2493-2494.

[16] Starfield B, Shi L, Macinko J. Contribution of primary care to health systems and health. Milbank Q. 2005;83(3):457-502.

[17] Furman D, Campisi J, Verdin E, et al. Chronic inflammation in the etiology of disease across the life span. Nat Med. 2019;25(12):1822-1832.

[18] Wallace DC. A mitochondrial paradigm of metabolic and degenerative diseases, aging, and cancer. Annu Rev Genet. 2005;39:359-407.

[19] Picard M, Wallace DC, Bhattacharyya S. The rise of mitochondria in medicine. Mitochondrion. 2016;30:105-116.

[20] Naviaux RK, Naviaux JC, Li K, et al. Metabolic features of chronic fatigue syndrome. Proc Natl Acad Sci U S A. 2016;113(37):E5472-E5480.

[21] Mills EL, Kelly B, O'Neill LAJ. Mitochondria are the powerhouses of immunity. Nat Immunol. 2017;18(5):488-498.

[22] Medzhitov R. Origin and physiological roles of inflammation. Nature. 2008;454(7203):428-435.

[23] Iliff JJ, Wang M, Liao Y, et al. A paravascular pathway facilitates CSF flow through the brain parenchyma and the clearance of interstitial solutes, including amyloid beta. Sci Transl Med. 2012;4(147):147ra111.

[24] Patti ME, Corvera S. The role of mitochondria in the pathogenesis of type 2 diabetes. Endocr Rev. 2010;31(3):364-395.

[25] Libby P, Ridker PM, Hansson GK. Progress and challenges in translating the biology of atherosclerosis. Nature. 2011;473(7347):317-325.

[26] Brown DA, Perry JB, Allen ME, et al. Mitochondrial function as a therapeutic target in heart failure. Nat Rev Cardiol. 2017;14(4):238-250.

[27] Davidson A, Diamond B. Autoimmune diseases. N Engl J Med. 2001;345(5):340-350.

[28] Magistretti PJ, Allaman I. A cellular perspective on brain energy metabolism and functional imaging. Neuron. 2015;86(4):883-901.

[29] Xie L, Kang H, Xu Q, et al. Sleep drives metabolite clearance from the adult brain. Science. 2013;342(6156):373-377.

[30] Tinetti ME, Bogardus ST Jr, Agostini JV. Potential pitfalls of disease-specific guidelines for patients with multiple conditions. N Engl J Med. 2004;351(27):2870-2874.

[31] Golomb BA, Evans MA. Statin adverse effects: a review of the literature and evidence for a mitochondrial mechanism. Am J Cardiovasc Drugs. 2008;8(6):373-418.

[32] Freedberg DE, Kim LS, Yang YX. The risks and benefits of long-term use of proton pump inhibitors: expert review and best practice advice from the American Gastroenterological Association. Gastroenterology. 2017;152(4):706-715.

[33] Listing J, Gerhold K, Zink A. The risk of infections is associated with rheumatoid arthritis, with its comorbidity and treatment. Rheumatology. 2013;52(1):53-61.

[34] Hyman M. The UltraMind Solution: Fix Your Broken Brain by Healing Your Body First. New York, NY: Scribner; 2009.

[35] Pasteur L. Germ Theory and Its Applications to Medicine and Surgery. Paris: Comptes Rendus de l'Académie des Sciences; 1878.

[36] Bernard C. An Introduction to the Study of Experimental Medicine. New York, NY: Dover Publications; 1957.

[37] Moberg CL. René Dubos: Friend of the Good Earth. Washington, DC: ASM Press; 2005.

[38] Sender R, Fuchs S, Milo R. Revised estimates for the number of human and bacteria cells in the body. PLoS Biol. 2016;14(8):e1002533.

[39] Casadevall A, Pirofski LA. Host-pathogen interactions: basic concepts of microbial commensalism, colonization, infection, and disease. Infect Immun. 2000;68(12):6511-6518.

[40] Rich PR. The molecular machinery of Keilin's respiratory chain. Biochem Soc Trans. 2003;31(Pt 6):1095-1105.

[41] Chandel NS. Mitochondria as signaling organelles. BMC Biol. 2014;12:34.

[42] Vander Heiden MG, Cantley LC, Thompson CB. Understanding the Warburg effect: the metabolic requirements of cell proliferation. Science. 2009;324(5930):1029-1033.

[43] Zhang Q, Raoof M, Chen Y, et al. Circulating mitochondrial DAMPs cause inflammatory responses to injury. Nature. 2010;464(7285):104-107.

[44] Cheng SY, Leonard JL, Davis PJ. Molecular aspects of thyroid hormone actions. Endocr Rev. 2010;31(2):139-170.

[45] Decrock E, Vinken M, De Vuyst E, et al. Connexin-related signaling in cell death: to live or let die? Cell Death Differ. 2009;16(4):524-536.

[46] Janeway CA Jr, Medzhitov R. Innate immune recognition. Annu Rev Immunol. 2002;20:197-216.

[47] Bonilla FA, Oettgen HC. Adaptive immunity. J Allergy Clin Immunol. 2010;125(2 Suppl 2):S33-S40.

[48] Sakaguchi S, Yamaguchi T, Nomura T, Ono M. Regulatory T cells and immune tolerance. Cell. 2008;133(5):775-787.

[49] Josefowicz SZ, Lu LF, Rudensky AY. Regulatory T cells: mechanisms of differentiation and function. Annu Rev Immunol. 2012;30:531-564.

[50] López-Armada MJ, Riveiro-Naveira RR, Vaamonde-García C, Valcárcel-Ares MN. Mitochondrial dysfunction and the inflammatory response. Mitochondrion. 2013;13(2):106-118.

[51] Levick JR, Michel CC. Microvascular fluid exchange and the revised Starling principle. Cardiovasc Res. 2010;87(2):198-210.

[52] Trevaskis NL, Kaminskas LM, Porter CJ. From sewer to saviour - targeting the lymphatic system to promote drug exposure and activity. Nat Rev Drug Discov. 2015;14(11):781-803.

[53] Girard JP, Moussion C, Förster R. HEVs, lymphatics and homeostatic immune cell trafficking in lymph nodes. Nat Rev Immunol. 2012;12(11):762-773.

[54] Zawieja DC. Contractile physiology of lymphatics. Lymphat Res Biol. 2009;7(2):87-96.

[55] Nedergaard M. Garbage truck of the brain. Science. 2013;340(6140):1529-1530.

[56] Cutler DM, Rosen AB, Vijan S. The value of medical spending in the United States, 1960-2000. N Engl J Med. 2006;355(9):920-927.

[57] Krumholz HM. The new cardiovascular risk factors: does their value differ in primary and secondary prevention? Cardiol Clin. 2001;19(3):317-326.

[58] Qaseem A, Wilt TJ, Kansagara D, et al. Hemoglobin A1c targets for glycemic control with pharmacologic therapy for nonpregnant adults with type 2 diabetes mellitus. Ann Intern Med. 2018;168(8):569-576.

[59] Bodenheimer T, Chen E, Bennett HD. Confronting the growing burden of chronic disease: can the US health care workforce do the job? Health Aff (Millwood). 2009;28(1):64-74.

[60] Aitken M, Kleinrock M. Medicine Use and Spending in the US. IQVIA Institute Report; 2023.

[61] Salami JA, Warraich H, Valero-Elizondo J, et al. National trends in statin use and expenditures in the US adult population from 2002 to 2013. JAMA Cardiol. 2017;2(1):56-65.

[62] Abramson JD, Rosenberg HG, Jewell N, Wright JM. Should people at low risk of cardiovascular disease take a statin? BMJ. 2013;347:f6123.

[63] American Diabetes Association. Economic costs of diabetes in the US in 2022. Diabetes Care. 2023;46(1):154-161.

[64] Hallberg SJ, McKenzie AL, Williams PT, et al. Effectiveness and safety of a novel care model for the management of type 2 diabetes at 1 year. Diabetes Ther. 2018;9(2):583-612.

[65] Katz DL, Meller S. Can we say what diet is best for health? Annu Rev Public Health. 2014;35:83-103.

[66] Barnett K, Mercer SW, Norbury M, et al. Epidemiology of multimorbidity and implications for health care, research, and medical education. Lancet. 2012;380(9836):37-43.

[67] Guthrie B, Makubate B, Hernandez-Santiago V, Dreischulte T. The rising tide of polypharmacy and drug-drug interactions. BMC Med. 2015;13:74.

[68] Mawe GM, Hoffman JM. Serotonin signalling in the gut - functions, dysfunctions, and therapeutic targets. Nat Rev Gastroenterol Hepatol. 2013;10(8):473-486.

[69] Greenhalgh T, Howick J, Maskrey N. Evidence based medicine: a movement in crisis? BMJ. 2014;348:g3725.

[70] Sertkaya A, Wong HH, Jessup A, Beleche T. Key cost drivers of pharmaceutical clinical trials in the United States. Clin Trials. 2016;13(2):117-126.

[71] Lexchin J, Bero LA, Djulbegovic B, Clark O. Pharmaceutical industry sponsorship and research outcome and quality. BMJ. 2003;326(7400):1167-1170.

[72] Bekelman JE, Li Y, Gross CP. Scope and impact of financial conflicts of interest in biomedical research. JAMA. 2003;289(4):454-465.

[73] Naci H, Brugts JJ, Fleurence R, Ades AE. Comparative effects of statins on major cerebrovascular events: a multiple-treatments meta-analysis of placebo-controlled and active-comparator trials. QJM. 2013;106(4):299-306.

[74] Godlee F. We want raw data, now. BMJ. 2016;355:i5770.

[75] Centers for Disease Control and Prevention. Prevalence of prediabetes among adults. MMWR Morb Mortal Wkly Rep. 2023;72(43):1156-1161.

[76] Boyle JP, Thompson TJ, Gregg EW, et al. Projection of the year 2050 burden of diabetes in the US adult population. Popul Health Metr. 2010;8:29.

[77] Rao Kondapally Seshasai S, Kaptoge S, Thompson A, et al. Diabetes mellitus, fasting glucose, and risk of cause-specific death. N Engl J Med. 2011;364(9):829-841.

[78] Kahn SE, Hull RL, Utzschneider KM. Mechanisms linking obesity to insulin resistance and type 2 diabetes. Nature. 2006;444(7121):840-846.

[79] Lowell BB, Shulman GI. Mitochondrial dysfunction and type 2 diabetes. Science. 2005;307(5708):384-387.

[80] Brownlee M. Biochemistry and molecular cell biology of diabetic complications. Nature. 2001;414(6865):813-820.

[81] Petersen KF, Dufour S, Befroy D, et al. Impaired mitochondrial activity in the insulin-resistant offspring of patients with type 2 diabetes. N Engl J Med. 2004;350(7):664-671.

[82] Grundy SM, Cleeman JI, Daniels SR, et al. Diagnosis and management of the metabolic syndrome. Circulation. 2005;112(17):2735-2752.

[83] Alberti KG, Eckel RH, Grundy SM, et al. Harmonizing the metabolic syndrome. Circulation. 2009;120(16):1640-1645.

[84] Deanfield JE, Halcox JP, Rabelink TJ. Endothelial function and dysfunction: testing and clinical relevance. Circulation. 2007;115(10):1285-1295.

[85] Ginsberg HN, Zhang YL, Hernandez-Ono A. Metabolic syndrome: focus on dyslipidemia. Obesity (Silver Spring). 2006;14 Suppl 1:41S-49S.

[86] Wilding JPH, Batterham RL, Calanna S, et al. Once-weekly semaglutide in adults with overweight or obesity. N Engl J Med. 2021;384(11):989-1002.

[87] Hall KD, Heymsfield SB, Kemnitz JW, et al. Energy balance and its components: implications for body weight regulation. Am J Clin Nutr. 2012;95(4):989-994.

[88] DeFronzo RA. From the triumvirate to the ominous octet: a new paradigm for the treatment of type 2 diabetes mellitus. Diabetes. 2009;58(4):773-795.

[89] Hotamisligil GS. Inflammation and metabolic disorders. Nature. 2006;444(7121):860-867.

[90] Taylor R. Calorie restriction and reversal of type 2 diabetes. Expert Rev Endocrinol Metab. 2016;11(6):521-528.

[91] Lean MEJ, Leslie WS, Barnes AC, et al. Primary care-led weight management for remission of type 2 diabetes (DiRECT): an open-label, cluster-randomised trial. Lancet. 2018;391(10120):541-551.

[92] DuBroff R, de Lorgeril M. Cholesterol confusion and statin controversy. World J Cardiol. 2015;7(7):404-409.

[93] Ravnskov U, de Lorgeril M, Diamond DM, et al. LDL-C does not cause cardiovascular disease: a comprehensive review of the current literature. Expert Rev Clin Pharmacol. 2018;11(10):959-970.

[94] World Health Organization. Cardiovascular diseases (CVDs). WHO Fact Sheets. Published 2021.

[95] Ford ES, Ajani UA, Croft JB, et al. Explaining the decrease in US deaths from coronary disease, 1980-2000. N Engl J Med. 2007;356(23):2388-2398.

[96] Sidney S, Quesenberry CP Jr, Jaffe MG, et al. Recent trends in cardiovascular mortality in the United States and public health goals. JAMA Cardiol. 2016;1(5):594-599.

[97] Sachdeva A, Cannon CP, Deedwania PC, et al. Lipid levels in patients hospitalized with coronary artery disease. Am Heart J. 2009;157(1):111-117.

[98] Keys A. Seven Countries: A Multivariate Analysis of Death and Coronary Heart Disease. Cambridge, MA: Harvard University Press; 1980.

[99] Ravnskov U. The Cholesterol Myths: Exposing the Fallacy that Saturated Fat and Cholesterol Cause Heart Disease. Washington, DC: New Trends Publishing; 2000.

[100] Ravnskov U, Diamond DM, Hama R, et al. Lack of an association or an inverse association between low-density-lipoprotein cholesterol and mortality in the elderly. BMJ Open. 2016;6(6):e010401.

[101] Petretta M, Costanzo P, Perrone-Filardi P, Chiariello M. Impact of gender in primary prevention of coronary heart disease with statin therapy. J Am Coll Cardiol. 2010;55(11):1135-1143.

[102] Kendrick M. The Great Cholesterol Con: The Truth About What Really Causes Heart Disease and How to Avoid It. London: John Blake Publishing; 2007.

[103] Steinberg D, Witztum JL. Oxidized low-density lipoprotein and atherosclerosis. Arterioscler Thromb Vasc Biol. 2010;30(12):2311-2316.

[104] Ridker PM, Danielson E, Fonseca FA, et al. Rosuvastatin to prevent vascular events in men and women with elevated C-reactive protein. N Engl J Med. 2008;359(21):2195-2207.

[105] Barth E, Stämmler G, Speiser B, Schaper J. Ultrastructural quantitation of mitochondria and myofilaments in cardiac muscle from 10 different animal species. J Mol Cell Cardiol. 1992;24(7):669-681.

[106] Rosca MG, Hoppel CL. Mitochondrial dysfunction in heart failure. Heart Fail Rev. 2013;18(5):607-622.

[107] Littarru GP, Langsjoen P. Coenzyme Q10 and statins: biochemical and clinical implications. Mitochondrion. 2007;7 Suppl:S168-S174.

[108] Ghirlanda G, Oradei A, Manto A, et al. Evidence of plasma CoQ10-lowering effect by HMG-CoA reductase inhibitors. Mol Aspects Med. 1997;18 Suppl:S137-S144.

[109] Silver MA, Langsjoen PH, Szabo S, et al. Effect of atorvastatin on left ventricular diastolic function. Am J Cardiol. 2004;93(2):259-261.

[110] Thompson PD, Panza G, Zaleski A, Taylor B. Statin-associated side effects. J Am Coll Cardiol. 2016;67(20):2395-2410.

[111] Kluge MA, Fetterman JL, Vita JA. Mitochondria and endothelial function. Circ Res. 2013;112(8):1171-1188.

[112] Hansson GK, Hermansson A. The immune system in atherosclerosis. Nat Immunol. 2011;12(3):204-212.

[113] Martel C, Li W, Fullerton B, et al. Lymphatic vasculature mediates macrophage reverse cholesterol transport in mice. J Clin Invest. 2013;123(4):1571-1579.

[114] Ornish D, Scherwitz LW, Billings JH, et al. Intensive lifestyle changes for reversal of coronary heart disease. JAMA. 1998;280(23):2001-2007.

[115] Estruch R, Ros E, Salas-Salvadó J, et al. Primary prevention of cardiovascular disease with a Mediterranean diet supplemented with extra-virgin olive oil or nuts. N Engl J Med. 2018;378(25):e34.

[116] Fiuza-Luces C, Garatachea N, Berger NA, Lucia A. Exercise is the real polypill. Physiology. 2013;28(5):330-358.

[117] Steptoe A, Kivimäki M. Stress and cardiovascular disease. Nat Rev Cardiol. 2012;9(6):360-370.

[118] Cappuccio FP, Cooper D, D'Elia L, et al. Sleep duration predicts cardiovascular outcomes. Eur Heart J. 2011;32(12):1484-1492.

[119] American Autoimmune Related Diseases Association. Autoimmune disease statistics. AARDA. Published 2023.

[120] Hayter SM, Cook MC. Updated assessment of the prevalence, spectrum and case definition of autoimmune disease. Autoimmun Rev. 2012;11(10):754-765.

[121] Fairweather D, Frisancho-Kiss S, Rose NR. Sex differences in autoimmune disease from a pathological perspective. Am J Pathol. 2008;173(3):600-609.

[122] Somers EC, Thomas SL, Smeeth L, Hall AJ. Are individuals with an autoimmune disease at higher risk of a second autoimmune disorder? Am J Epidemiol. 2009;169(6):749-755.

[123] Gabriel SE, Crowson CS, Kremers HM, et al. Survival in rheumatoid arthritis: a population-based analysis of trends over 40 years. Arthritis Rheum. 2003;48(1):54-58.

[124] Klein L, Kyewski B, Allen PM, Hogquist KA. Positive and negative selection of the T cell repertoire: what thymocytes see (and don't see). Nat Rev Immunol. 2014;14(6):377-391.

[125] Mueller DL. Mechanisms maintaining peripheral tolerance. Nat Immunol. 2010;11(1):21-27.

[126] Cusick MF, Libbey JE, Fujinami RS. Molecular mimicry as a mechanism of autoimmune disease. Clin Rev Allergy Immunol. 2012;42(1):102-111.

[127] Guilherme L, Kalil J. Rheumatic fever and rheumatic heart disease: cellular mechanisms leading autoimmune reactivity and disease. J Clin Immunol. 2010;30(1):17-23.

[128] Fasano A. Leaky gut and autoimmune diseases. Clin Rev Allergy Immunol. 2012;42(1):71-78.

[129] Arrieta MC, Bistritz L, Meddings JB. Alterations in intestinal permeability. Gut. 2006;55(10):1512-1520.

[130] Mu Q, Kirby J, Reilly CM, Luo XM. Leaky gut as a danger signal for autoimmune diseases. Front Immunol. 2017;8:598.

[131] Bischoff SC, Barbara G, Buurman W, et al. Intestinal permeability - a new target for disease prevention and therapy. BMC Gastroenterol. 2014;14:189.

[132] Theofilopoulos AN, Kono DH, Baccala R. The multiple pathways to autoimmunity. Nat Immunol. 2017;18(7):716-724.

[133] Miller SD, Vanderlugt CL, Begolka WS, et al. Persistent infection with Theiler's virus leads to CNS autoimmunity via epitope spreading. Nat Med. 1997;3(10):1133-1136.

[134] Angelin A, Gil-de-Gómez L, Dahber S, et al. Foxp3 reprograms T cell metabolism to function in low-glucose, high-lactate environments. Cell Metab. 2017;25(6):1282-1293.

[135] Smolen JS, Aletaha D, McInnes IB. Rheumatoid arthritis. Lancet. 2016;388(10055):2023-2038.

[136] Mercer LK, Lunt M, Low AL, et al. Risk of solid cancer in patients exposed to anti-tumour necrosis factor therapy. Ann Rheum Dis. 2015;74(6):1086-1093.

[137] Konijeti GG, Kim N, Lewis JD, et al. Efficacy of the autoimmune protocol diet for inflammatory bowel disease. Inflamm Bowel Dis. 2017;23(11):2054-2060.

[138] Marras C, Beck JC, Bower JH, et al. Prevalence of Parkinson's disease across North America. NPJ Parkinsons Dis. 2018;4:21.

[139] Wallin MT, Culpepper WJ, Campbell JD, et al. The prevalence of MS in the United States. Neurology. 2019;92(10):e1029-e1040.

[140] Petersen RC. Mild cognitive impairment as a diagnostic entity. J Intern Med. 2004;256(3):183-194.

[141] Camandola S, Mattson MP. Brain metabolism in health, aging, and neurodegeneration. EMBO J. 2017;36(11):1474-1492.

[142] Swerdlow RH, Burns JM, Khan SM. The Alzheimer's disease mitochondrial cascade hypothesis. J Alzheimers Dis. 2010;20 Suppl 2:S265-S279.

[143] Schapira AH. Mitochondria in the aetiology and pathogenesis of Parkinson's disease. Lancet Neurol. 2008;7(1):97-109.

[144] Campbell GR, Worrall JT, Mahad DJ. The central role of mitochondria in axonal degeneration in multiple sclerosis. Mult Scler. 2014;20(14):1806-1813.

[145] de la Monte SM, Wands JR. Alzheimer's disease is type 3 diabetes - evidence reviewed. J Diabetes Sci Technol. 2008;2(6):1101-1113.

[146] Heneka MT, Kummer MP, Latz E. Innate immune activation in neurodegenerative disease. Nat Rev Immunol. 2014;14(7):463-477.

[147] Salter MW, Stevens B. Microglia emerge as central players in brain disease. Nat Med. 2017;23(9):1018-1027.

[148] Hansen DV, Hanson JE, Bhanu M. Microglia in Alzheimer's disease. J Cell Biol. 2018;217(2):459-472.

[149] Perry VH, Holmes C. Microglial priming in neurodegenerative disease. Nat Rev Neurol. 2014;10(4):217-224.

[150] Biessels GJ, Staekenborg S, Brunner E, Brayne C, Scheltens P. Risk of dementia in diabetes mellitus. Lancet Neurol. 2006;5(1):64-74.

[151] Gorelick PB, Scuteri A, Black SE, et al. Vascular contributions to cognitive impairment and dementia. Stroke. 2011;42(9):2672-2713.

[152] Ferro JM, Caeiro L, Figueira ML. Neuropsychiatric sequelae of stroke. Nat Rev Neurol. 2016;12(5):269-280.

[153] Shokri-Kojori E, Wang GJ, Wiers CE, et al. Beta-amyloid accumulation in the human brain after one night of sleep deprivation. Proc Natl Acad Sci U S A. 2018;115(17):4483-4488.

[154] Shi L, Chen SJ, Ma MY, et al. Sleep disturbances increase the risk of dementia: a systematic review and meta-analysis. Sleep Med Rev. 2018;40:4-16.

[155] Yaffe K, Laffan AM, Harrison SL, et al. Sleep-disordered breathing, hypoxia, and risk of mild cognitive impairment and dementia. JAMA. 2011;306(6):613-619.

[156] DiSabato DJ, Quan N, Bhatt AP. Neuroinflammation: the devil is in the details. J Neurochem. 2016;139 Suppl 2:136-153.

[157] Da Mesquita S, Fu Z, Bhattacharyya D. Meningeal lymphatics affect microglia responses and anti-Aβ immunotherapy. Nature. 2021;593(7858):255-260.

[158] Ngandu T, Lehtisalo J, Solomon A, et al. A 2 year multidomain intervention of diet, exercise, cognitive training, and vascular risk monitoring versus control. Lancet. 2015;385(9984):2255-2263.

[159] Bredesen DE. Reversal of cognitive decline: a novel therapeutic program. Aging (Albany NY). 2014;6(9):707-717.

[160] Institute of Medicine. Beyond Myalgic Encephalomyelitis/Chronic Fatigue Syndrome: Redefining an Illness. Washington, DC: National Academies Press; 2015.

[161] Wolfe F, Clauw DJ, Fitzcharles MA, et al. The American College of Rheumatology preliminary diagnostic criteria for fibromyalgia. Arthritis Care Res (Hoboken). 2010;62(5):600-610.

[162] Jason LA, Benton MC, Valentine L, et al. The economic impact of ME/CFS: individual and societal costs. Dyn Med. 2008;7:6.

[163] Pendergrast T, Brown A, Sunnquist M, et al. Housebound versus nonhousebound patients with myalgic encephalomyelitis and chronic fatigue syndrome. Chronic Illn. 2016;12(4):292-307.

[164] Komaroff AL, Fagioli LR, Doolittle TH, et al. Health status in patients with chronic fatigue syndrome and in general population and disease comparison groups. Am J Med. 1996;101(3):281-290.

[165] Naviaux RK. Perspective: Cell danger response biology - the new science that connects environmental health with mitochondria and the rising tide of chronic illness. Mitochondrion. 2020;51:40-45.

[166] Fluge Ø, Mella O, Bruland O, et al. Metabolic profiling indicates impaired pyruvate dehydrogenase function in myalgic encephalopathy/chronic fatigue syndrome. JCI Insight. 2016;1(21):e89376.

[167] Naviaux RK. Metabolic features and regulation of the healing cycle - a new model for chronic disease pathogenesis and treatment. Mitochondrion. 2019;46:278-297.

[168] Rasa S, Nora-Krukle Z, Henning N, et al. Chronic viral infections in myalgic encephalomyelitis/chronic fatigue syndrome (ME/CFS). J Transl Med. 2018;16(1):268.

[169] Missailidis D, Annesley SJ, Fisher PR. Pathological mechanisms underlying myalgic encephalomyelitis/chronic fatigue syndrome. Diagnostics (Basel). 2019;9(3):80.

[170] Serhan CN. Pro-resolving lipid mediators are leads for resolution physiology. Nature. 2014;510(7503):92-101.

[171] Weller RO, Djuanda E, Yow HY, Carare RO. Lymphatic drainage of the brain and the pathophysiology of neurological disease. Acta Neuropathol. 2009;117(1):1-14.

[172] Clauw DJ. Fibromyalgia: a clinical review. JAMA. 2014;311(15):1547-1555.

[173] Woolf CJ. Central sensitization: implications for the diagnosis and treatment of pain. Pain. 2011;152(3 Suppl):S2-S15.

[174] Ji RR, Nackley A, Huh Y, Terrando N, Bhargava A. Neuroinflammation and central sensitization in chronic and widespread pain. Anesthesiology. 2018;129(2):343-366.

[175] Tomas C, Brown A, Strassheim V, et al. Cellular bioenergetics is impaired in patients with chronic fatigue syndrome. PLoS One. 2017;12(10):e0186802.

[176] Hornig M, Montoya JG, Klimas NG, et al. Distinct plasma immune signatures in ME/CFS are present early in the course of illness. Sci Adv. 2015;1(1):e1400121.

[177] Louveau A, Smirnov I, Keyes TJ, et al. Structural and functional features of central nervous system lymphatic vessels. Nature. 2015;523(7560):337-341.

[178] Castro-Marrero J, Sáez-Francàs N, Santillo D, Alegre J. Treatment and management of chronic fatigue syndrome/myalgic encephalomyelitis: all roads lead to Rome. Br J Pharmacol. 2017;174(5):345-369.

[179] Reckeweg HH. Homotoxicology: Illness and Healing Through Anti-homotoxic Therapy. Albuquerque, NM: Menaco Publishing; 1984.

[180] Littarru GP, Tiano L. Clinical aspects of coenzyme Q10: an update. Nutrition. 2010;26(3):250-254.

[181] Martin LR, Williams SL, Haskard KB, DiMatteo MR. The challenge of patient adherence. Ther Clin Risk Manag. 2005;1(3):189-199.

[182] Jornayvaz FR, Shulman GI. Regulation of mitochondrial biogenesis. Essays Biochem. 2010;47:69-84.

[183] Lozupone CA, Stombaugh JI, Gordon JI, Jansson JK, Knight R. Diversity, stability and resilience of the human gut microbiota. Nature. 2012;489(7415):220-230.

[184] Cramer SC, Sur M, Bhardwaj A, et al. Harnessing neuroplasticity for clinical applications. Brain. 2011;134(Pt 6):1591-1609.

[185] Farber DL, Yudanin NA, Restifo NP. Human memory T cells: generation, compartmentalization and homeostasis. Nat Rev Immunol. 2014;14(1):24-35.

[186] Genuis SJ. Elimination of persistent toxicants from the human body. Hum Exp Toxicol. 2011;30(1):3-18.

[187] Bland JS. The Disease Delusion: Conquering the Causes of Chronic Illness for a Healthier, Longer, and Happier Life. New York, NY: Harper Wave; 2014.

[188] Starfield B. Is US health really the best in the world? JAMA. 2000;284(4):483-485.

[189] Kresser C. Unconventional Medicine: Join the Revolution to Reinvent Healthcare, Reverse Chronic Disease, and Create a Practice You Love. Austin, TX: Lioncrest Publishing; 2017.

[190] Nicolson GL, Gan R, Haier J. Multiple co-infections (Mycoplasma, Chlamydia, human herpes virus-6) in blood of chronic fatigue syndrome patients. APMIS. 2003;111(5):557-566.

[191] van der Kolk BA. The Body Keeps the Score: Brain, Mind, and Body in the Healing of Trauma. New York, NY: Penguin Books; 2014.

[192] Chrousos GP. Stress and disorders of the stress system. Nat Rev Endocrinol. 2009;5(7):374-381.

[193] Lord RS, Bralley JA. Laboratory Evaluations for Integrative and Functional Medicine. 2nd ed. Duluth, GA: Metametrix Institute; 2008.

[194] Munnich A, Rotig A, Chretien D, Saudubray JM, Cormier V, Rustin P. Clinical presentations and laboratory investigations in respiratory chain deficiency. Eur J Pediatr. 1996;155(4):262-274.

[195] Marc DT, Ailts JW, Campeau DC, Bull MJ, Olson KL. Neurotransmitters excreted in the urine as biomarkers of nervous system activity. Neurosci Biobehav Rev. 2011;35(3):635-644.

[196] Frosst P, Blom HJ, Milos R, et al. A candidate genetic risk factor for vascular disease: a common mutation in methylenetetrahydrofolate reductase. Nat Genet. 1995;10(1):111-113.

[197] Selhub J. Folate, vitamin B12 and vitamin B6 and one carbon metabolism. J Nutr Health Aging. 2002;6(1):39-42.

[198] Vighi G, Marcucci F, Sensi L, Di Cara G, Frati F. Allergy and the gastrointestinal system. Clin Exp Immunol. 2008;153 Suppl 1:3-6.

[199] Qin J, Li R, Raes J, et al. A human gut microbial gene catalogue established by metagenomic sequencing. Nature. 2010;464(7285):59-65.

[200] Roseth AG, Fagerhol MK, Aadland E, Schjonsby H. Assessment of the neutrophil dominating protein calprotectin in feces. Scand J Gastroenterol. 1992;27(9):793-798.

[201] Fasano A. Zonulin, regulation of tight junctions, and autoimmune diseases. Ann N Y Acad Sci. 2012;1258(1):25-33.

[202] Canani RB, Costanzo MD, Leone L, Pedata M, Meli R, Calignano A. Potential beneficial effects of butyrate in intestinal and extraintestinal diseases. World J Gastroenterol. 2011;17(12):1519-1528.

[203] Sampson HA, Aceves S, Bock SA, et al. Food allergy: a practice parameter update - 2014. J Allergy Clin Immunol. 2014;134(5):1016-1025.

[204] Vojdani A. For the assessment of intestinal permeability, size matters. Altern Ther Health Med. 2013;19(1):12-24.

[205] Catassi C, Bai JC, Bonaz B, et al. Non-celiac gluten sensitivity: the new frontier of gluten related disorders. Nutrients. 2013;5(10):3839-3853.

[206] Freitag FM, Cestari TF. What causes dark circles under the eyes? J Cosmet Dermatol. 2007;6(3):211-215.

[207] Genuis SJ. Sensitivity-related illness: the escalating pandemic of allergy, food intolerance and chemical sensitivity. Sci Total Environ. 2010;408(24):6047-6061.

[208] Heaton KW, Radvan J, Cripps H, Mountford RA, Braddon FE, Hughes AO. Defecation frequency and timing, and stool form in the general population. Gut. 1992;33(6):818-824.

[209] Schnakenberg E, Fabig KR, Stanulla M, et al. A cross-sectional study of self-reported chemical-related sensitivity is associated with gene variants of drug-metabolizing enzymes. Environ Health. 2007;6:6.

[210] Hibbard JH, Greene J. What the evidence shows about patient activation: better health outcomes and care experiences. Health Aff (Millwood). 2013;32(2):207-214.

[211] Crinnion WJ. The CDC fourth national report on human exposure to environmental chemicals: what it tells us about our toxic burden. Altern Med Rev. 2010;15(2):101-109.

[212] Chikly B. Silent Waves: Theory and Practice of Lymph Drainage Therapy. 2nd ed. Scottsdale, AZ: IHH Publishing; 2004.

[213] Sears ME, Kerr KJ, Bray RI. Arsenic, cadmium, lead, and mercury in sweat: a systematic review. J Environ Public Health. 2012;2012:184745.

[214] Mesnage R, Clair E, Gress S, Then C, Szekacs A, Seralini GE. Cytotoxicity on human cells of Cry1Ab and Cry1Ac Bt insecticidal toxins alone or with a glyphosate-based herbicide. J Appl Toxicol. 2013;33(7):695-699.

[215] DiNicolantonio JJ, O'Keefe JH. Omega-6 vegetable oils as a driver of coronary heart disease: the oxidized linoleic acid hypothesis. Open Heart. 2018;5(2):e000898.

[216] Kessler R. Studies begin to clarify health risks from common chemical. Environ Health Perspect. 2015;123(2):A42.

[217] Mortimer PS, Rockson SG. New developments in clinical aspects of lymphatic disease. J Clin Invest. 2014;124(3):915-921.

[218] Popkin BM, D'Anci KE, Rosenberg IH. Water, hydration, and health. Nutr Rev. 2010;68(8):439-458.

[219] Shields JW. Lymph, lymph glands, and homeostasis. Lymphology. 1992;25(4):147-153.

[220] Olszewski WL. Contractility patterns of normal and pathologically changed human lymphatics. Ann N Y Acad Sci. 2002;979:52-63.

[221] Vairo GL, Miller SJ, McBrier NM, Buckley WE. Systematic review of efficacy for manual lymphatic drainage techniques in sports medicine and rehabilitation. J Man Manip Ther. 2009;17(3):e80-e89.

[222] Ballatori N, Krance SM, Notenboom S, Shi S, Tieu K, Hammond CL. Glutathione dysregulation and the etiology and progression of human diseases. Biol Chem. 2009;390(3):191-214.

[223] Silbergeld EK, Patrick TE. Environmental exposures, toxicologic mechanisms, and adverse pregnancy outcomes. Am J Obstet Gynecol. 2005;192(5 Suppl):S11-S21.

[224] Petschow BW, Burnett B, Shaw AL, Weaver EM, Klein GL. Serum-derived bovine immunoglobulin/protein isolate: postulated mechanism of action for management of enteropathy. Clin Exp Gastroenterol. 2014;7:181-190.

[225] Schieber M, Bhardwaj N. Resolution of inflammation: basic concepts and relevance for disease. Cold Spring Harb Perspect Med. 2018;8(2):a024034.

[226] Spite M, Claria J, Serhan CN. Resolvins, specialized proresolving lipid mediators, and their potential roles in metabolic diseases. Cell Metab. 2014;19(1):21-36.

[227] Fernandez DC, Fogerson PM, Lazzerini Ospri L, et al. Light affects mood and learning through distinct retina-brain pathways. Cell. 2018;175(1):71-84.e18.

[228] Nieman DC, Wentz LM. The compelling link between physical activity and the body's defense system. J Sport Health Sci. 2019;8(3):201-217.

[229] Besedovsky L, Lange T, Haack M. The sleep-immune crosstalk in health and disease. Physiol Rev. 2019;99(3):1325-1380.

[230] Cole SW, Capitanio JP, Chun K, Arevalo JM, Ma J, Cacioppo JT. Myeloid differentiation architecture of leukocyte transcriptome dynamics in perceived social isolation. Proc Natl Acad Sci U S A. 2015;112(49):15142-15147.

[231] Leipner J, Saller R. Systemic enzyme therapy in oncology: effect and mode of action. Drugs. 2000;59(4):769-780.

[232] Gupta SC, Patchva S, Aggarwal BB. Therapeutic roles of curcumin: lessons learned from clinical trials. AAPS J. 2013;15(1):195-218.

[233] Dröge W, Breitkreutz R. Glutathione and immune function. Proc Nutr Soc. 2000;59(4):595-600.

[234] Warburg O. On the origin of cancer cells. Science. 1956;123(3191):309-314.

[235] Bianco AC, Kim BW. Deiodinases: implications of the local control of thyroid hormone action. J Clin Invest. 2006;116(10):2571-2579.

[236] Hood DA, Memme JM, Oliveira AN, Triolo M. Maintenance of skeletal muscle mitochondria in health, exercise, and aging. Annu Rev Physiol. 2019;81:19-41.

[237] Cannon B, Nedergaard J. Brown adipose tissue: function and physiological significance. Physiol Rev. 2004;84(1):277-359.

[238] de Cabo R, Mattson MP. Effects of intermittent fasting on health, aging, and disease. N Engl J Med. 2019;381(26):2541-2551.

[239] Laukkanen JA, Laukkanen T, Kunutsor SK. Cardiovascular and other health benefits of sauna bathing: a review of the evidence. Mayo Clin Proc. 2018;93(8):1111-1121.

[240] Kirkland JL, Tchkonia T. Senolytic drugs: from discovery to translation. J Intern Med. 2020;288(5):518-536.

[241] Pettegrew JW, Levine J, McClure RJ. Acetyl-L-carnitine physical-chemical, metabolic, and therapeutic properties. Mol Psychiatry. 2000;5(6):616-632.

[242] Littarru GP, Tiano L. Bioenergetic and antioxidant properties of coenzyme Q10: recent developments. Mol Biotechnol. 2007;37(1):31-37.

[243] Kennedy DO. B vitamins and the brain: mechanisms, dose and efficacy - a review. Nutrients. 2016;8(2):68.

[244] Pilchova I, Klacanova K, Tatarkova Z, Kaplan P, Racay P. The involvement of Mg2+ in regulation of cellular and mitochondrial functions. Oxid Med Cell Longev. 2017;2017:6797460.

[245] Mari M, Morales A, Colell A, Garcia-Ruiz C, Fernandez-Checa JC. Mitochondrial glutathione, a key survival antioxidant. Antioxid Redox Signal. 2009;11(11):2685-2700.

[246] Bredesen DE. The End of Alzheimer's: The First Program to Prevent and Reverse Cognitive Decline. New York, NY: Avery; 2017.

[247] Raichle ME, Gusnard DA. Appraising the brain's energy budget. Proc Natl Acad Sci U S A. 2002;99(16):10237-10239.

[248] Daneman R, Prat A. The blood-brain barrier. Cold Spring Harb Perspect Biol. 2015;7(1):a020412.

[249] Cobley JN, Fiorello ML, Bailey DM. 13 reasons why the brain is susceptible to oxidative stress. Redox Biol. 2018;15:490-503.

[250] Lee H, Xie L, Yu M, et al. The effect of body posture on brain glymphatic transport. J Neurosci. 2015;35(31):11034-11044.

[251] Hastings MH, Maywood ES, Brancaccio M. Generation of circadian rhythms in the suprachiasmatic nucleus. Nat Rev Neurosci. 2018;19(8):453-469.

[252] Gooley JJ, Chamberlain K, Smith KA, et al. Exposure to room light before bedtime suppresses melatonin onset and shortens melatonin duration in humans. J Clin Endocrinol Metab. 2011;96(3):E463-E472.

[253] Bonaz B, Bazin T, Pellissier S. The vagus nerve at the interface of the microbiota-gut-brain axis. Front Neurosci. 2018;12:49.

[254] Gerritsen RJS, Band GPH. Breath of life: the respiratory vagal stimulation model of contemplative activity. Front Hum Neurosci. 2018;12:397.

[255] Ebrahim IO, Shapiro CM, Williams AJ, Fenwick PB. Alcohol and sleep I: effects on normal sleep. Alcohol Clin Exp Res. 2013;37(4):539-549.

[256] Slutsky I, Abumaria N, Wu LJ, et al. Enhancement of learning and memory by elevating brain magnesium. Neuron. 2010;65(2):165-177.

[257] Aoyama K, Nakaki T. Impaired glutathione synthesis in neurodegeneration. Int J Mol Sci. 2013;14(10):21021-21044.

[258] Guo S, Bhardwaj A, Bhardwaj N. The biology of tissue repair: from wound healing to regeneration. Nat Rev Mol Cell Biol. 2020;21(12):729-743.

[259] Longo VD, Panda S. Fasting, circadian rhythms, and time-restricted feeding in healthy lifespan. Cell Metab. 2016;23(6):1048-1059.

[260] Ames BN. Low micronutrient intake may accelerate the degenerative diseases of aging through allocation of scarce micronutrients by triage. Proc Natl Acad Sci U S A. 2006;103(47):17589-17594.

[261] Holick MF. The vitamin D deficiency pandemic: approaches for diagnosis, treatment and prevention. Rev Endocr Metab Disord. 2017;18(2):153-165.

[262] Khatri M, Naughton RJ, Clifford T, Harper LD, Corr L. The effects of collagen peptide supplementation on body composition, collagen synthesis, and recovery from joint injury and exercise: a systematic review. Amino Acids. 2021;53(10):1493-1506.

[263] Buettner D, Skemp S. Blue Zones: lessons from the world's longest lived. Am J Lifestyle Med. 2016;10(5):318-321.

www.ingramcontent.com/pod-product-compliance
Lightning Source LLC
Chambersburg PA
CBHW071430230926
51846CB00001B/170
* 9 7 8 1 9 7 1 4 4 9 0 4 3 *